T0215504

Dementia in Prison

This innovative volume exposes dementia as a condition that the aging prison population is increasingly facing. Going beyond exploring the need to understand dementia within prison populations, it argues that health and social care professionals and prison staff must ensure that older prisoners are screened and assessed for dementia, diagnosed and provided with the appropriate care and support.

Dementia in Prison covers three key areas: healthcare services in prison settings and how these affect the rapidly aging prison population; the human rights of prisoners with dementia, alongside the ethics of healthcare in this environment; and the current state of support for prisoners with dementia and recommendations for future assessment, diagnosis and policies.

This provocative book will be invaluable to scholars in the fields of public health, social work, criminology and medical sociology as well as healthcare professionals, including nurses and prison staff.

Joanne Brooke is a professor of nursing, and director of the Centre of Social Care, Health and Related Research, and the Institute for Dementia and Culture Collaborative. Joanne is a qualified adult nurse and chartered health psychologist. Her main areas of research include topics related to equity of care and hard-to-research groups; acute community and prison care and support for people with dementia, delirium and stroke; explorations of the implementation of theory into practice to provide evidence-based care; and elements of undergraduate curriculum development with regard to dementia, delirium, research and transgender health. Joanne supervises undergraduate and postgraduate students, including both PhD students and those completing a professional doctorate in health psychology.

Routledge Studies in Public Health

www.routledge.com/Routledge-Studies-in-Public-Health/book-series/
RSPH

Available titles include:

Conceptualising Public Health
Historical and Contemporary Struggles over Key Concepts
Edited by Johannes Kananen, Sophy Bergenheim, Merle Wessel

Global Health and Security
Critical Feminist Perspectives
Edited by Colleen O'Manique and Pieter Fourie

Women's Health and Complementary and Integrative Medicine
Edited by Jon Adams, Amie Steel, Alex Broom and Jane Frawley

Managing the Global Health Response to Epidemics
Social Science Perspectives
Edited by Mathilde Bourrier, Nathalie Brender and Claudine Burton-Jeangros

The Anthropology of Tobacco
Ethnographic Adventures in Non-Human Worlds
Edited by Mathilde Bourrier, Nathalie Brender and Claudine Burton-Jeangros

Public Health Evaluation and the Social Determinants of Health
Kelley Allyson

Sustainable Sexual Health
Analysing the Implementation of the SDGs
Tony Sandset, Eivind Engebretsen and Kirstin Heggen

Dementia in Prison
An Ethical Framework to Support Research, Practice and Prisoners
Edited by Joanne Brooke

Dementia in Prison

An Ethical Framework to Support Research, Practice and Prisoners

Edited by Joanne Brooke

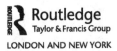

LONDON AND NEW YORK

First published 2021
by Routledge
2 Park Square, Milton Park, Abingdon, Oxon OX14 4RN

and by Routledge
52 Vanderbilt Avenue, New York, NY 10017

Routledge is an imprint of the Taylor & Francis Group, an informa business

British Library Cataloguing-in-Publication Data
A catalogue record for this book is available from the British Library

Library of Congress Cataloging-in-Publication Data
A catalog record for this book has been requested

ISBN: 978-0-367-25917-4 (hbk)
ISBN: 978-0-429-29104-3 (ebk)

Typeset in Bembo
by Apex CoVantage, LLC

To my Mum, an inspiration for so many, the most amazing woman I had the privilege to call 'Mum', her journey through dementia has and always will influence everything I do.

Contents

Figures

Tables

Contributors

Lydia Aston is a postdoctoral researcher in the Centre for Social Care, Health and Related Research at Birmingham City University. Lydia is experienced in conducting health research and has a particular interest in using qualitative methods to understand the illness experiences of individuals living with neurological, life-limiting conditions and those in palliative care. Lydia has worked in dementia research, specifically focusing on medication management for people living with dementia from both a social care perspective and in the community. She is also interested in applying phenomenological research to a variety of clinical settings where interventions can be guided by the importance of subjective meanings and lived experience in directing healthcare. Lydia is a health psychologist in training.

Melindy Brown is a lecturer in criminology and deputy course leader of Criminology, Policing & Investigation, and Security Studies at Birmingham City University. Her main areas of research are around the topics of desistance, rehabilitation, substance use, prisons and probation. Melindy has a bachelor's (Honours) and a master's (Honours) in criminology. She is currently completing her PhD, with a focus on support within the community to encourage desistance from offending and substance misuse, particularly alcohol-related offending. Additionally, Melindy is a prison befriender for the New Bridge Foundation, a befriending service between members of the public and people in prison.

Monika Rybacka is an assistant professor in nursing and dementia lead at Coventry University. Her main areas of research are mental health nursing and dementia care; specialising in the use of meaningful activities in dementia care, prisoners and dementia and student nurse and post-graduate education in dementia care. Monika has a Diploma of Higher Education in mental health nursing, a bachelor's (Honours) degree in psychology and health science and a postgraduate diploma in healthcare management. She is currently completing her clinical doctorate at Stirling University, with a focus on how nurses receive and use support in acute hospital settings to provide care for people living with dementia. Monika is also the secretary and a board member for the Institute for Dementia and Culture Collaborative and a member of Sigma Theta Tau International Honor Society of Nursing.

1　An aging prison population

Melindy Brown and Joanne Brooke

The rapidly increasing aging prison population

Many countries across the world are seeing an increase in the average age of those in prison, with older prisoners the fastest-growing group within prison populations. Because of this trend, prison services are required to address a number of emerging issues that previously were not prevalent in the younger prison population. The first section in this chapter will put these figures into context in prison systems within England and Wales, the United States of America (USA) and Australia.

England and Wales

In England and Wales, the prison estate is split into separate prisons that accommodate one of three groups – adult males, young people and women (Grimwood, 2015). On 13 March 2020, there were 83,917 people in prison, across the adult and young offender institution prison estate in England and Wales (Ministry of Justice et al., 2020). Prison population figures within the Prison Service for England and Wales remain high, with their admissions to prison being the second highest in Western Europe at a rate of 140 per 100,000 of the national population, only being outweighed by Scotland (World Prison Brief and Institute for Crime & Justice Policy Research, 2019). High prison numbers alone put the prison estate under immense pressure; however, this is further stretched when it is noted that a number of those who are incarcerated are considered to be older prisoners.

Within the Prison Service of England and Wales, the age of the prison population has grown over time. Between 2002 and 2013, there was an increase of 100 per cent of those aged 50 to 59, and an increase of 120 per cent of those over 60 years old, making these age ranges the first and second fastest-growing groups respectively (House of Commons Justice Committee, 2013). In December 2017, the number of people aged 50 and over was 13,522, which was 16 per cent of the total adult prison population of those over 18 years old (Her Majesty's Inspectorate of Prisons and Care Quality Commission, 2018a). In a report predicting the prison population between 2017 and 2021, it was projected that prisoners over the age of 50 would increase in both absolute terms and as a proportion of the overall prison population (Ministry of Justice, 2017). In 2018, update figures suggested a projected 3.6 per cent increase: from 13,616 prisoners in June 2018 to 14,100 in June 2022 (Ministry of Justice, 2018).

Recent projection figures do suggest that the number of older prisons aged 50 and over will decline to 12,500 by 2023, in line with the prison population decrease (Ministry of Justice, 2019a). However, as this decline will be corresponding with the prison population's overall movement, it does not prevent the issues linked to having a high number of individuals within this population who would be considered older. Currently, 13,980 people within prison in England and Wales are aged 50 and over, which is equal to just under 20 per cent of the prison population (Ministry of Justice, 2019b). Of this figure, 5,157 are over 60 years old, and 1,813, are over 70 years old (Ministry of Justice, 2019b). As such, the past year's figures are currently aligning with the previous projections that predicted an increase.

United States of America

The United States of America is another country experiencing an aging prison population. The prison system in the USA, due to the size of their geographical location is far bigger than England and Wales. The population of the USA accounts for approximately 5 per cent of the world's population, but in terms of prisoners, holds nearly 25 per cent of the world's prison population (The Osborne Association, 2018). Therefore, it is not surprising that the USA incarcerates the largest number of people per capita than any other nation, at a rate of 698 per 100,000 residents (Sawyer and Wagner, 2019). To put this into context, it is important to consider how many people are in prison within the USA and within what types of prison. Terminology is important at this point, as jails refer to short-term facilities, whereas prisons are facilitated by the Federal Bureau of Prisons or by the state and are used as long-term facilities for those who have been sentenced.

> The American criminal justice system holds almost 2.3 million people in 1,719 state prisons, 109 federal prisons, 1,772 juvenile correctional facilities, 3,163 local jails, and 80 Indian Country jails as well as in military prisons, immigration detention facilities, civil commitment centers, state psychiatric hospitals, and prisons in the U.S. territories.
>
> (Sawyer and Wagner, 2019)

Similar to England and Wales, the prison population in the USA has increased over time. Between 2000 and 2009, there was a 79 per cent increase of those 55 and older entering the prison system (Williams et al., 2012). The incarceration of large numbers of older people still occurs, with older people encompassing the fastest-growing group in the USA's prison estate (Sharupski et al., 2018).

When excluding jails, and only including state and federal prisons, the number of prisoners over the age of 55 increased by 280 per cent between 1999 and 2016, in comparison to a 3 per cent growth of young adults (McKillop and Boucher, 2018). As a result, the older prison population in the USA has risen from 3 per cent to 11 percent of the total prison population (McKillop and Boucher, 2018). The rise in older people in prison has been projected to account for a third of USA's prison population by 2030 (The Osborne Association, 2018). This rise is likely to put an unsustainable pressure on the USA's justice system as a whole (The Osborne Association, 2018).

Australia

A further Western region worth noting when considering older people in prison is Australia. In comparison to England and Wales, and the USA, Australia has the least number of prisoners, at 43,028 in June 2019 (Australian Bureau of Statistics, 2019). Despite this, Australia has seen a dramatic increase in their incarceration rate. In 1990, the rate was 114 per 100,000 adults; in 2000, it was 152 per 100,000; and in 2010, 175 per 100,000 (Leigh, 2019). The most recent figures show Australia's national imprisonment rate is currently higher than England and Wales at 219 per 100,000 (Australian Bureau of Statistics, 2019). Furthermore, it has been found that in proportionate terms, Australia has seen a 130 per cent increase in incarceration rates between 1985 and 2018 (Leigh, 2019).

Among this increase in imprisonment rates, Australia has seen a similar trend to England and Wales, and the USA in that they have an aging prison population. Between 2001 and 2010, Australia's prison population aged 50 and over increased by 81.6 per cent, with a further increase of 67 per cent taking place between 2010 and 2018 (Johnstone, 2019). In June 2018, there were 5,554 incarcerated people aged 50 and over, and 1,156 aged 65 and over (Johnstone, 2019). When specifically looking at those aged 65 and older, the percentage increased between 2001 and 2010 to 128 per cent, and a further 119.4 per cent increase between 2010 and 2018 (Johnstone, 2019).

After having considered the statistics for the general prison populations, in comparison to the older prisoner population specifically, it is clear that England and Wales, the USA and Australia are all seeing an increase in those prisoners often referred to as older. Later on in this chapter, we address continuing discussions regarding what constitutes an older prisoner. However, beforehand, it is important to recognise what factors could be exacerbating the aging prison population across the three Western regions.

Contributing factors to the aging prison population

When discussing the contributing factors for the aging prison population, it is important to compare and align these factors with the global context. Worldwide, there is an aging population, with the World Health Organization and the US National Institute of Aging (2011) projecting that the number of people over the age of 65 will grow from approximately 524 million in 2010 (representing 8 per cent of the world's population) to 1.5 billion in 2050 (representing 16 per cent of the world's population). When considering the number of people over the age of 60, it is expected that by 2050 they will account for 22 per cent of the world's population, outweighing the number of children aged under five years old (World Health Organization, 2018). In England and Wales, the USA and Australia, the 'baby boomer generation', one of the largest generations, will soon all be over the age of 60, and as such these countries are now entering a period of significant increase in their older population.

The Prison Service of England and Wales is separate from the rest of the United Kingdom (UK); however, when discussing general population demographics, the findings often discuss England and Wales within the remit of the UK. The UK has been noted to have an aging population (Office for National Statistics, 2018), with just under 12 million people aged 65 and over (Age UK, 2019a), and it is estimated that by 2030, those aged 65 and over will account for approximately 33 per cent of the population (Office for National Statistics, 2017). In the USA, projections suggest that for the first time in the nation's history, in 2034, adults aged 65 and over will outnumber those under the age of 18 (Medina et al., 2020). In 2015, the median age of the Australian population was 37.2, slightly lower than the USA at 37.6 and the UK at 40.2 (United Nations, 2017). Nevertheless, in 2015, the percentage of those 65 and older in Australia was the same as the USA at 15 per cent and similar to the UK at 18 per cent (United Nations, 2017). Furthermore, Australia's projection on growth is similar to the UK and USA, with the proportion of adults 65 and over expected to increase to 22 per cent of the population by 2057 and 25 per cent by 2097 (Australian Bureau of Statistics, 2014).

Alongside the growing number of older people in the general populations of England and Wales, the USA and Australia, these regions are tough on crime and apply imprisonment as a dominant method of punishment (Newburn, 2007; National Research Council, 2014; Mackay, 2015). Therefore, it is likely this has an impact on the number of older people entering prison. To understand this in more depth, it is important to consider the legal systems in each of these countries in terms of the types of sentencing, and how they affect older people in the criminal justice system.

Sentencing in England and Wales

The sentencing guidelines for England and Wales continue to evolve to address rising crime rates, such as the introduction of custodial sentences for breaches of bail (Sentencing Council, 2018). In the absence of the death penalty, the most severe sanction in England and Wales is very long terms in prison (Prison Reform Trust, 2019), and it is commonplace for prisoners to serve 10 years or longer. The Prison Service of England and Wales has the highest number of prisoners serving a life sentence in Europe (Crewe et al., 2019). The average tariff for a mandatory life sentence, excluding those on a whole-life tariff, has increased from 12.5 years in 2003 to 21.3 years in 2016 (Prison Reform Trust, 2019).

The Prison Service of England and Wales implemented indeterminate sentences; although these were abolished in 2012, there are still 11,025 prisoners (15 per cent of the sentenced prison population) serving an indeterminate sentence (Ministry of Justice, 2019b). This figure includes prisoners serving an indeterminate imprisonment for public protection (IPP) sentence (Ministry of Justice, 2019b). The IPP sentence, in a similar manner to life sentences, requires offenders to serve a minimum tariff before the parole board decides if they can be released due to their risk to public safety (The Howard League for Penal Reform, 2016). Currently, 2,223 prisoners serving an IPP sentence have yet to be released, with 90 per cent having completed their minimum sentence (Ministry of Justice, 2019b). The difficulty arises due to the need to demonstrate a prisoner is no longer a risk to society, which enhances the chances of longer prison sentences. The rate of recalls for prisoners serving an IPP sentence also outweighs those being released (Ministry of Justice, 2019b). A third of prisoners serving an IPP sentence are aged 50 or over; therefore, people are growing old within prison, with the number of those aged 60 and over tripling in 15 years (Ministry of Justice, 2019c). An important element for consideration is 90 per cent of prisoners 80 years old and over were sentenced to prison when they were 70 years old and over (House of Lords, 2017a).

The aging prison population is further enhanced due to the type of crimes committed by older prisoners, as long sentences for serious sexual and violent crimes have significantly increased (Prison Reform Trust, 2019). Within the prison population of those aged 50 and over, 45 per cent have been convicted for a sexual offence, and 23 per cent for a violent offence against another person (House of Lords, 2017b). Furthermore, within the population of prisoners aged 80 and over, 87 per cent were convicted for a sexual offence (Ministry of Justice, 2017). Because of the high levels of social stigma attached to both sexual and violent crimes, harsher and longer sentences have been implemented to address societal concerns. Because of those societal pressures, there has also been an increased focus by the police and prosecutors to pursue sexual offences (Mann, 2012). Advances in forensic evidence as well as a greater societal awareness of historic sex offences, those which occurred several decades ago, have led to the increase in the number of potential older perpetrators being brought to trial (Yorston, 2015; Crawley and Sparks, 2005a). The combination of focused police and prosecution services, improved technology and enhanced investigative policing abilities has increased the number of older perpetrators being convicted and sentenced for sexual offences (Crawley and Sparks, 2005b).

Sentencing in the USA

Sentencing policies and practices in the USA have developed dramatically; during the 1930s to 1975, there was a focus on indeterminate sentencing, rehabilitation and parole release, with a move from 1975 to 1984 towards sentencing reform, focusing on determinate sentencing (Tonry, 2013) and retribution (Murphy, 1973; Morris, 1974; von Hirsch, 1976). However, the key sentencing changes that have affected the current system within the USA, particularly in relation to the increase of older prisoners, is the 'tough on crime' period from 1984 to 1996. Many of these policies are still in place today, including mandatory minimum sentences and life without parole and three-strikes laws (Sabol et al., 2002; Stemen et al., 2006). The three-strikes law involved the issue of a life sentence when an individual was convicted for their third offence. However, mandatory minimum sentences and life without parole sentences have had the main impact on the increasing older prison population within the USA prison systems.

Mandatory minimum sentencing laws require the courts to impose minimum sentences for certain crimes, reducing sentencing discretion by judicial actors (Nelson, 1992). The spike in the use of mandatory minimum sentences occurred after the Sentencing Reform Act 1984, whereby many federal crimes and drug-related state crimes had significant mandatory minimum sentencing. This has had a lasting impact on the number of people currently serving a mandatory minimum sentence. Recent figures have shown the number of people convicted of an offence that carries a mandatory minimum sentence has reduced since fiscal year 2010 (United States Sentencing Commission, 2017). Yet, this has not prevented the significant impact that mandatory minimum sentences ultimately continue to have on the size of the federal prison population (United States Sentencing Commission, 2017). Statistics from fiscal year 2016 show that around two-thirds of offenders on a mandatory minimum sentence received no relief from the penalty (United States Sentencing Commission, 2017).

Mandatory minimum sentencing is an important factor that has influenced the increase of older prisoners in the USA prison population (Yorston and Taylor, 2006). In 1994 and 2011, there was a persistent increase in violent offenders aged 50 and over (Kim and Peterson, 2014). In 2009, 25.8 per cent of prisoners aged 55 and over entering state prisons was due to violent offences, which was second only to drug offences (Bonczar et al., 2011). However, drug offences compared to other offences have remained significantly higher in receiving mandatory minimum sentences, although this has dropped from 91 per cent in 1990 to 67 per cent in 2016 (United States Sentencing Commission, 2017). However, it is worth noting that mandatory minimum sentences are not limited to violent offences, highlighting how these sentences further affect the aging prison population (Human Rights Watch, 2012). Nevertheless, severe sentencing laws that include mandatory minimum sentences, in addition to reductions in parole eligibility, inevitably increase the number of people in prison and the length of time they serve (Shahani, 2017; The Sentencing Project, 2017). Both these factors have an impact on the number of older prisoners who have aged in prison or those who have entered prison at a later age.

The life sentences have had a significant impact on the aging prison population in the USA. The US rate of incarceration for life is 50 per 100,000, which is approximately equivalent to the incarceration rates of Denmark, Finland and Sweden combined (Gottschalk, 2012). Many nations have not embraced life without parole to the same extent as the USA (Leigey and Schartmueller, 2019) because '[a] sentence of life imprisonment without the possibility of parole is in many ways no more than a death sentence without an execution date' (Berry, 2010, p. 1112). In 2016, 206,268 prisoners were serving a life sentence (the equivalent of 1 in 7 prisoners), with 44,311 prisoners serving a virtual life sentence of 50 years or longer (The Sentencing Project, 2017). Both types of life with parole sentences and life without parole sentences have increased since 1984; however, there remains significantly more life without parole sentences (The Sentencing Project, 2017). In 2016, 53,290 prisoners (1 in 28 prisoners) were serving a life without parole sentence (The Sentencing Project, 2017). Despite the size of the USA, just under 53 per cent of those people serving a sentence of life without parole were disproportionately distributed across Florida, Pennsylvania, California, Louisiana and the federal system (The Sentencing Project, 2017).

Sentencing in Australia

Crime rates in Australia have declined, whilst the prison population has increased, because of changes in the justice and sentencing practices and policies, including the use of mandatory sentences (Senate Legal and Constitutional Affairs Committee, 2013). Much of this is because of the change in legislation, including reduced judicial discretion, which has again been driven by the approach of being 'tough on crime' (Cunneen et al., 2016). In the Northern Territory, Queensland and South Australia, mandatory sentencing can be fixed or minimum sentences, or attached to a specific crime, such as mandatory life sentences (Deckert and Sarre, 2017). The introduction of fixed or minimum sentences by Australian Parliaments reduces judicial discretion and increases the severity of punishments (Gray and Elmore, 2012). All states and territories within Australia have mandatory sentences, with the types of offences receiving a mandatory sentence varying. For example, mandatory sentences will be imposed for repeat offenders of residential burglary in Western Australia, for murder and rape in the Northern Territory, for murder of a police officer in New South Wales, for child sex offences in Queensland, for intentional or reckless gross violence in Victoria and for certain people smuggling offences in the Commonwealth (Law Council of Australia, 2014). Furthermore, older individuals in Australian prisons serving sentences for offences that receive lengthy sentences, such as sex- and drug-related offences (Grant, 1999; Potter et al., 2007), are likely to be further affected by mandatory sentences.

In some Australian jurisdictions, both parole and probation officers have internal guidelines imposed on them that require all breaches of parole to be reported, regardless of the severity of the breach. These policies particularly affect those who lack financial, housing and relationship support (Senate Legal and Constitutional Affairs Committee, 2013). In some jurisdictions, people who breach their parole forfeit their time spent in the community and must serve the remainder of their sentence, from the time they were initially released, as such increasing the length of their original full-term sentence (Bartels and Freiberg, 2019). These two aspects have left parole and probation officers reluctant to recommend release on parole because of the implications and likelihood of a breach (Senate Legal and Constitutional Affairs Committee, 2013). As such, the overall impact is higher numbers of people either remaining in, or returning to, prison. Older prisoners are less likely to reoffend; however, due to their more serious offences (Potter et al., 2007), in addition to an averseness to promote parole and community alternatives (Kerbs and Jolley, 2009), the prison population continues to age.

The third important factor is recidivism, which is the tendency of a convicted criminal to reoffend. The high rates of recidivism affect the Australian prison population (Dunn, 2017), as 54.2 per cent of prisoners released during 2017 and 2018 returned to corrective services. Although this figure varies slightly by territories, in the years 2015 and 2016, South Australia had a rate of 37.1 per cent; Victoria, 43.7 per cent; and the Northern Territory, 55.9 per cent (Australian Government Productivity Commission, 2019). In 2016, New South Wales had the highest state prison population, with 48 per cent of prisoners returning within two years (Olding, 2016). Recidivism, mandatory minimums and limiting options for parole have all contributed to the aging prison population within Australia (Aday, 2006; Dawes, 2009; Grant, 1999; Kempker, 2003; Kerbs and Jolley, 2009; Potter et al., 2007).

The contributing factors to aging prison populations across England and Wales, USA and Australia are the age of individuals when entering prison, the type of sentence they have received and mandatory minimum sentences, as older prisoners tend to be convicted of crimes with long prison sentences, alongside younger prisoners serving lengthy and indeterminate sentences.

Defining the older prisoner

First, a number of distinctions between older and younger prisoners are important to recognise. In the England and Wales Prison Service, older prisoners are less likely to have formal education (46 per cent) than those aged 21–49 (68 per cent). Second, there is a correlation between older male prisoners and their convicted offence. Older prisoners are more likely to be serving a sentence for sexual offences; this accounts for 46 per cent of convictions of male prisoners over the age of 50 and increases significantly to 79 per cent of male prisoners over the age of 70 (HM Prison and Probation Service, 2018). Third, 60 per cent of older prisoners reported their current prison sentence as their first, compared to 45 per cent of younger prisoners (Omolade, 2014).

Recently, the definition of an older prisoner in the UK has begun to be operationalised across different institutions, bodies and charities. For example HM Inspectorate of Prisons (2008), the Prison Reform Trust and Age UK (2019) recognise and define an older prisoner as someone aged 50 or older. The HM Prison and Probation Service (2018) has also recently applied this definition, following the House of Commons Justice Committee's fifth report of session 2013–2014, where evidence was submitted from RECOOP (Resettlement and Care of Older ex-Offenders and Prisoners), Age UK, Restore Support Network and the Prison Reform Trust. The evidence presented included both the negative impact of prison on a prisoner's physical and mental health and previous addictions and/or homelessness, which accelerated the prisoner's physical aging and declining health. These and further evidence to support the definition of an older prisoner will be discussed later.

The significance of an accurate definition of an older prisoner is important, as the HM Prison and Probation Service (2018) in their model of operational delivery have identified older prisoners as a specialist cohort. This model supports the delivery of the three main functions of England and Wales prisons, which involves reception, training and resettlement, to ensure each prison meets the needs of their specialist cohorts, both comprehensively and effectively, including older prisoners' complex needs. Therefore, it is essential that the definition of the older person is evidence-based and represents the negative impact of prison on prisoner's physical and mental well-being as well as their health and social care needs, as the definition informs both policy and practice.

One of the key critiques that is discussed within the debate of defining older prisoners is the argument of chronological age versus functionality and ability. Defining prisoners by their chronological age of 50 and over is due to the accelerated aging process that enhances their likelihood of developing disabilities and chronic illnesses at an earlier age than those within the general population (Williams et al., 2012). A clear and significant difference between the health of prisoners and that of the general population has been identified. In 1999, Grant identified a 10-year differential between a prisoner's chronological age and physiological health and of those living in the community, due to deficiencies both prior and within in prison (Trotter and Baidawi, 2015).

Because of the accelerated aging that is linked to the prison experience, prisoners who are aged 50 and over in the UK are referred to as older prisoners (Age UK, 2019b); this is similar to the regulation of some states within the USA (Williams, 2006). However, a number of states in the USA base their definition on a prisoner's degree of disability, rather than chronological age (Anno et al., 2004). The Australian Bureau of Statistics (2009) defined older people as those aged 65 or over. However, a report by Baidawi et al., (2011) established that in practise, the age of 50 and over is applied as a functional definition for older prisoners (Grant, 1999; Kerbs and Jolley, 2009; Stojkovic, 2007). Currently, there is no global consensus or definition of an older prisoner. However, this is important to determine in order to support the development of relevant policies relating to prison and healthcare services for older people.

The terminology of 'older prisoner' relates to the prisoners' chronological age, but there are also several types of older prisoners who need to be considered when applying this term. One classification of older prisoners identifies three distinct populations: prisoners entering prison for the first time over the age of 50, recidivist prisoners (who have been in and out of prison throughout their life) and prisoners who are serving long sentences and grow old within prison (Baidawi et al., 2011). A further classification of older prisoners identifies two distinct populations with prisoners entering prison for the first time over the age of 50, by defining the length of their sentence, including those who serve short-terms and long-terms. Long-term older prisoners were also identified as being more likely to be sentenced for historic sexual or violent crimes (American Civil Liberties Union, 2012).

The different classifications of older prisoners are important; however, the extreme levels of stress experienced by all older prisoners is unquestionable (Stojkovic, 2007). Older prisoners as a collective are also more likely to have faced disadvantages throughout their life, on the basis of their demographic background, substance misuse, poor societal relationships, financial difficulties and health problems. In Australia and the USA, it is important to also explore the impact of ethnicity, for example prisoners from an indigenous or first nations background are often classified as older prisoners in terms of their functionality, despite their age being chronologically younger (Baidawi et al., 2011). In England and Wales, prisoners from black, Asian and minority ethnic background have been found to have more negative experiences of prison because of less support with their health needs and higher levels of discrimination across the prison estate (Lammy Report, 2017). It is clear that ethnicity is a particular individual factor that can lead to disproportionalities in terms of health, and as such the need for more flexibility in defining older prisoners.

Because of the impact of prison on aging, there needs to be a recognition that the health and social needs of prisoners should be considered as complex from a younger age, as their level of functionality may not correspond with their chronological age. The next section explores the health and social needs of older prisoners.

Health and social needs of older prisoners

Prisoners are acknowledged to have an accelerated aging process compared to the general public, and this is more pronounced in older prisoners. This section will commence with an exploration of older prisoners' health and the risks and patterns of increased chronic illnesses, followed by a section exploring the contributing factors to the development of these conditions. The final section will focus on the social needs of older prisoners and the current barriers and challenges of supporting these needs in prisons in the Prison Service of England and Wales.

Increased chronic illness

In England and Wales, the prevalence of long-term chronic (LTC) diseases in older prisoners has been explored and estimated in a number of representative samples of older prisoners (Hayes et al., 2012; Omolade, 2014). A study completed in the North West of England estimated LTC diseases to range from 71 per cent in those aged 50 to 54 to 92 per cent in those over the age of 70 (Hayes et al., 2012). In a longitudinal cohort study conducted by the Ministry of Justice, 59 per cent of prisoners over the age of 50 reported an LTC disease or disability, compared to 27 per cent of younger prisoners (Omolade, 2014). HM Prison and Probation Service (2018) identified 50 per cent of older prisoners who reported an LTC disease actually reported three or more different LTC diseases. Similarly, within prisons in Switzerland, older prisoners were 2.26 times more likely to report an LTC disease compared to younger prisoners, and older prisoners were on average likely to report 4.27 LTC diseases compared to 1.62 reported by younger prisoners (Wangmo et al., 2015).

LTC diseases encompass both physical and mental health; in the North of England, 50 per cent of older prisoners entering prison presented with clinical signs of depression, which was associated with unmet physical health needs (O'Hara et al., 2016). In German prisons, older prisoners were identified as having a higher rate of suicide than those in the community of the same age (Opitz-Welke et al., 2019). Older prisoners have been identified to be at a higher risk of depression, psychosis, bipolar disorder, dementia, cognitive impairment, personality disorder and anxiety disorders than older people living in the community (Di Lorito et al., 2018). In the UK, the most prominent physical illnesses of older prisoners include osteoarthritis (35 per cent), asthma (17 per cent), hypertension (32 per cent), diabetes (19 per cent), hearing loss (21 per cent) and ischemic heart disease (18 per cent) (Hayes et al., 2012). A review of published data from the US identified older prisoners had higher rates of diabetes mellitus, liver disease and cardiovascular conditions, and higher rates of depression, anxiety and suicidal ideation, although no empirical data on cognitive impairment or dementia among older prisoners was identified; however, this review did identify that 20 per cent of the older prisoners required support to meet their activities of daily living (Sharupski et al., 2018).

Older prisoners' LTC diseases can affect their functional abilities, such as being able to meet their activities of daily living, which prevent them from being independent whilst in prison. Multi-morbidity patterns and their association with functional limitations of older prisoners have been explored (Gates et al., 2018). Three patterns of illnesses were identified: first, chronic diseases such as diabetes, hypertension, dyslipidaemia (high cholesterol) and cardiovascular disease, of which 60.3 per cent of the population within this study had at least one, and 34.3 per cent more than three; second, geriatric conditions, such as joint problems, dementia and fractures, of which 70 per cent had at least one, 23.4 per cent two, and 6.1 per cent three; and third, substance misuse and mental health disorders, including neurological conditions, such as epilepsy and headaches, of which 61.3 per cent had at least one, and 20.3 per cent more than three (Gates et al., 2018). The impact of three or more chronic diseases or one geriatric condition was related to a significant risk of functional impairment, whereas substance misuse and mental health disorders were not related to functional impairment (Gates et al., 2018). However, it was noted that 48.4 per cent of the population under study had conditions across all three patterns of illnesses, and age was the only variable that was a significant risk factor for functional impairment (Gates et al., 2018).

Contributing factors to poor health

The remainder of this section will explore the elements that contribute to prisoners' accelerated aging, especially among older prisoners, and this will include poor health and life choices before and during a prison sentence, significant trauma, grief and loss, alongside the complex interplay of poor health, complex health needs, social disadvantage and lower levels of education. Poor health and lifestyle choices include the use of alcohol and drugs. A review of 13 studies identified the prevalence of alcohol abuse and dependence on admission to prison ranged from 18 to 30 per cent, whereas estimates of drug abuse and dependence ranged from 10 to 40 per cent (Fazel et al., 2006). Regarding significant trauma, grief and loss, including childhood adversities, prisoners are more likely than their community-dwelling peers to have experienced interpersonal loss, significant family problems, abuse and neglect (Schnittker et al., 2012). Childhood adversities have also been associated with the development of poor health behaviours and mental health disorders in later life (Non et al., 2016; Green et al., 2010).

The roles of social disadvantage and crime and their impact on health remain a continued debate, although those who work closely with prisoners would not deny the majority come from socially disadvantaged backgrounds. Social disadvantage encompasses the comparative lack of social and economic resources. One explanation of the impact of social disadvantage is that it is only moderately related to crime involvement; the significant element is childhood disadvantage, when young people are exposed to both criminal activity and poor health behaviour choices (Wilkstrom and Treiber, 2016). Lower levels of education have been associated with a higher risk of unemployment and inconsistent job histories, which can be demonstrated as problematic as over a half of the prisoners in this category reported being fired at least once from a job (Visher et al., 2004). A low level of education prior to incarceration has also been identified to be negatively associated with increased health problems, although education whilst in prison can mitigate this effect (Nowotny et al., 2016).

Social needs of older prisoners

Social care needs of older people have often been described through their inability to independently maintain their own activities of daily living (ADL).

In the community, 10 activities of daily living are described: bathing, grooming, toilet use, transfer (from bed to chair), feeding, dressing, mobility, stairs, bowels and bladder control. A common assessment to determine an individual's level of ADL functioning is the Barthel Index (Mahoney and Barthel, 1965; Collin et al., 2008), which is commonly used in clinical practice and is sensitive to either improvement or decline in a person's ADL functioning. The application of the Barthel Index remains a relevant assessment of disability in the prison setting, although in the USA, Prison ADL (PADL) have been developed (Williams, 2006). PADL include functional activities specifically related to American prison systems and regimes, such as dropping to the floor for alarms, walking to the hall for meals, standing in line for medications and climbing on and off a top bunk. These are applicable ADL for prisoners in the USA system as they address issues that may be modifiable, such as being placed on a low bunk, but may not be applicable to other systems around the world.

In England and Wales, the Prison Service Instruction (PSI) for Adult Social Care (National Offender Management Service, 2015) provides criteria for prisoners who have two or more social care needs, which if unmet are likely to affect their well-being significantly. A number of these criteria are related to prisoner's ADL and include managing and maintaining nutrition, personal hygiene, toilet needs, being appropriately clothed, being able to use the prison safely, maintaining a habitable cell, developing relationships and accessing activities. Public Health England (2017) suggests prison establishments should be viewed as providers of social care, as they already include the provision of meals, laundry services, education and exercise for the prisoners who are temporarily living there. Therefore, social care to support the physical needs of prisoners has to be included and provided jointly by health services, social services and prison services; in the UK, this includes volunteer services such as Age UK. Social care teams support prisoners on a day-to-day basis with physical health needs, although other interventions, such as informal peer support systems, namely the Gold Coats or Buddies (further explained in Chapter 4), provide informal low levels of social care support.

The assessment of social needs of older prisoners is essential to identify prisoners who have difficulties in maintaining certain ADL, such walking on uneven surfaces or stairs. In England and Wales, the Independent Monitoring Board (2017) recognised areas in some prisons remained inaccessible to prisoners with mobility issues, which in some cases included healthcare provision, and many prisons were still unable to support prisoners with mobility problems (HM Chief Inspector of Prisons, 2019). The built environment of prisons in England and Wales has been recognised as a barrier to supporting prisoners with their social care needs (HM Inspectorate of Prison and Care Quality Commission, 2018b). Furthermore, it is essential to address those needs of older prisoners, as unmet social needs are associated with depression and increased suicidal ideation (Barry et al., 2017).

A prominent social need of older prisoners is that of socialisation with peers; because of increased isolation through imprisonment and prison regimes that do not support older prisoners or those with disabilities to leave their cells during the day, the impact of being locked in their cells for the majority of the day increases their social isolation and loneliness (Enggist et al., 2014; Hayes et al., 2013; Joyce and Maschi, 2016). In the Prison Service of England and Wales, purposeful activity for older prisoners has begun to be implemented but remained inconsistent across prisons; the HM Chief Inspector of Prisons (2019) reported 'some good age-specific activities, however in other prisons no specific provision and little meaningful activity for those not at work'. These initiatives and others will be discussed in more depth in Chapter 4, although there is a need to acknowledge a lack of robust evaluations of social care practices in prisons for older prisoners and a lack of overarching programmes, models or guidelines (Senior et al., 2013; Tucker et al., 2017).

Although social needs of older prisoners have begun to be recognised, other elements also need to be considered, such as the negative impact of victimisation and bullying by younger prisoners (Fazel et al., 2016), the lack of knowledge and training of prison staff to support older prisoners (Brooke and Rybacka, 2020), alongside the unsuitable prison environments to support mobility of older prisoners around the prison and lack of meaningful and purposeful activities. All these factors negatively affect the social needs of older prisoners, leaving them prone to loneliness, isolation, anxiety and depression (Baidawi et al., 2016).

Summary

Throughout this chapter, what has become clear is that the Western World, particularly England and Wales, the USA and Australia, are being affected not only by an aging general population, but an aging prison population. Although people across the world are living longer, there are several other reasons that are affecting the growth of older prisoner population. There are similarities across the various regions that have clearly had an impact on this, particularly the move towards being 'tough on crime'. The use of mandatory minimum and indeterminate sentences have had a considerable influence on the length of time that individuals have spent in prison and as such, enhanced the number of older prisoners. Furthermore, older people have tended to be incarcerated for crimes that can hold long sentences, such as sex offences, violence and drug offences. Older people are often defined based on their chronological age; however, this chapter has highlighted that functionality and disadvantages within life can cause prisoners to develop physical and mental health conditions at a younger age. Older prisoners are also at a higher risk of LTC diseases than those living in the community because of poor health and life choices before and during a prison sentence, complex social disadvantages and lower levels of education. This chapter finishes with the importance of assessing the health and social needs of older prisoners to ensure prison environments and systems can meet their needs.

References

Aday, R. (2006). Ageing prisoners. In B. Berkman, S. D'Ambruoso (Eds.) *Handbook of Social Work in Health and Ageing*. Santa Barbara, CA: Oxford University Press.

Age UK (2019a). *Later Life in the United Kingdom 2019*. Available from: www.ageuk.org. uk/globalassets/age-uk/documents/reports-and publications/later_life_uk_factsheet.pdf [Accessed on: 19 March 2020].

Age UK (2019b). *Older Prisoners (England and Wales)*, July. Available from: www.ageuk.org. uk/globalassets/age-uk/documents/policy-positions/care-and-support/ppp_older_pris-oners_en_wa.pdf [Accessed on: 26 March 2020].

American Civil Liberties Union (2012). *At America's Expense. The Mass Incarceration of the Elderly*. Available from: www.aclu.org/sites/default/files/field_document/elderlyprison report_20120613_1.pdf [Accessed on: 20 March 2020].

Anno, B.J., Camilia, G., Lawrence, J.E., Shansky, R. (2004). *Correctional Health Care: Addressing the Needs of Elderly, Chronically Ill, and Terminally Ill Inmates*. Available from: https://nicic.gov/correctional-health-care-addressing-needs-elderly-chronically-ill-and-terminally-ill-inmates [Accessed on: 26 March 2020].

Australian Bureau of Statistics (2009). *Australian Social Trends: Future Population Growth and Ageing*, cat. no. 4102.0. Canberra: Australian Bureau of Statistics.

Australian Bureau of Statistics (2014). *Australian Historical Population Statistics, 2014*, cat. no. 3105.0.65.001. Canberra: Australian Bureau of Statistics.

Australian Bureau of Statistics (2019). 4517.0 – *Prisoners in Australia, 2019*, cat. no. 4517.0. Canberra: Australian Bureau of Statistics.

Australian Government Productivity Commission (2019). *Report on Government Services 2019*. Available from: www.pc.gov.au/research/ongoing/report-on-government-services/ 2019/justice#attachtables [Accessed on: 25 March 2020].

Baidawi, S., Trotter, C., O'Connor, D.W. (2016). An integrated exploration of factors associated with psychological distress among older prisoners. *The Journal of Forensic Psychiatry & Psychology*, 27: 815–834.

Baidawi, S., Turner, S., Trotter, C., Browning, C., Collier, P., O'Connor, D., Sheehan, R. (2011). Older prisoners – a challenge for Australian corrections. *Trends & Issues in Crime and Criminal Justice*, 426: 1–18.

Barry, L.C., Wakefield, D.B., Trestman, R.L., Conwell, Y. (2017). Disability in prison activities of daily living and likelihood of depression and suicidal activities in older prisoners. *International Journal of Psychiatry*, 32: 1141–1149.

Bartels, L., Freiberg, A. (2019). Street time is no sweet time: granting credit for time on parole in Australia. *Current Issues in Criminal Justice*, 31(4): 476–492.

Berry, W. (2010). More different than life, less different than death. *Ohio State Law Journal*, 71: 1109–1146.

Bonczar, T.P., Hughes, T.A., Wilson, D.J., Ditton, P.M. (2011). *National Corrections Reporting Program, 2009 – Statistical Tables, Bureau of Justice Statistics*. Available from: www.bjs.gov/ index.cfm?ty=pbdetail&iid=2174 [Accessed on: 23 March 2020].

Brooke, J., Rybacka, M. (2020). Development of a dementia education workshop for prison staff, prisoners, health and social care professionals. *Journal of Correctional Health Care*, DOI: 10.1177/1078345820916444.

Collin, C., Wade, D.T., Davies, S., Horne, V. (2008). The Barthel index. *Disability and Rehabilitation*, 10(2): 61–63.

Crawley, E., Sparks, R. (2005a). Hidden injuries? Researching the experiences of older men in English prisons. *Howard Journal of Criminal Justice*, 44(4): 345–356.

Crawley, E., Sparks, R. (2005b). Surviving the prison experience? Imprisonment and elderly men. *Prison Service Journal*, 160: 3–8.

Crewe, B., Hulley, S., Wright, S. (2019). *Life Imprisonment from Young Adulthood*. London: Palgrave Macmillan.

Cunneen, C., Baldry, E., Brown, D., Brown, M., Schwartz, M., Steel, A. (2016). *Penal Culture and Hyperincarceration: The Revival of the Prison*. Farnham: Ashgate.

Dawes, J. (2009). Ageing prisoners: issues for social work. *Australian Social Work*, 62(2): 258–271.

Deckert, A., Sarre, R. (2017). *The Palgrave Handbook of Australian and New Zealand Criminology, Crime and Justice*. Basingstoke: Palgrave Macmillan.

Di Lorito, C., Vollm, B., Dening, T. (2018). Psychiatric disorders among older prisoners: a systematic review and comparison study against older people in the community. *Aging and Mental Health*, 22(1): 1–10.

Dunn, I. (2017). *Chalk and Cheese: Australian vs. Norway*. Sydney: Community Justice Coalition.

Enggist, S., Møller, L., Galea, G., Udesen, C. (2014). *Prisons and Health. Copenhagen: World Health Organization Regional Office for Europe*. Available from: www.euro.who.int/__data/assets/pdf_file/0005/249188/Prisons-and-Health.pdf [Accessed on: 16 March 2020].

Fazel, S., Bains, P., Doll, H. (2006). Substance abuse and dependence in prisoners: a systematic review. *Addiction*, 101(2): 181–191.

Fazel, S., Hayes, A.J., Bartellas, K., Clerici, M., Trestman, R. (2016). Mental health of prisoners: prevalence, adverse outcomes, and interventions. *The Lancet Psychiatry*, 3(9): 871–881.

Gates, L.M., Hunter, E.G., Dicks, V., Jessa, P.N., Walker, V., Yoo, W. (2018). Multimorbidity patterns and associations with functional limitations among an aging prison population. *Archives of Gerontology and Geriatrics*, 77: 115–123.

Gottschalk, M. (2012). No way out? Life sentences and the politics of penal reform. In C. Ogletree, A. Sarat (Eds.) *Life Without Parole: America's New Death Penalty?* New York: New York University Press.

Grant, A. (1999). Elderly inmates: issues for Australia. *Trends & Issues in Crime and Criminal Justice*, no. 115. Canberra: Australian Institute of Criminology.

Gray, A., Elmore, G. (2012). The constitutionality of minimum mandatory sentencing regimes. *Journal of Judicial Administration*, 22(1): 37–47.

Green, J.G., McLaughlin, K.A., Berglund, P.A., Gruber, M.J., Sampson, N.A., Zaslavsky, A.M., Kessler, R.C. (2010). Childhood adversities and adult psychiatric disorders in the national comorbidity survey replication I: associations with first onset of DSMIV disorders. *Archives of General Psychiatry*, 67: 113–123.

Grimwood, G.G. (2015). *Categorisation of Prisoners in the UK*. Briefing Paper Number 07437, 29 December. London: House of Commons.

Hayes, A.J., Burns, A., Turnbull, P., Shaw, J.J. (2012). The health and social needs of older male prisoners. *International Journal of Geriatric Psychiatry*, 27: 1155–1162.

Hayes, A.J., Burns, A., Turnbull, P., Shaw, J.J. (2013). Social and custodial needs of older adults in prison. *Age and Ageing*, 42(5): 589–593.

Her Majesty's Chief Inspector of Prisons (2019). *Annual Report 2018–2019*. Available from: https://assets.publishing.service.gov.uk/government/uploads/system/uploads/attachment_data/file/814689/hmip-annual-report-2018-19.pdf [Accessed on: 16 March 2020].

Her Majesty's Inspectorate of Prisons (2008). *Older Prisoners in England and Wales: A Follow-up to the 2004 Thematic Review by HM Chief Inspector of Prisons*. Available from: www.justiceinspectorates.gov.uk/hmiprisons/wp-content/uploads/sites/4/2014/07/Older-Prisoners-2008-Follow-up-Thematic.pdf [Accessed on: 16 March 2020].

Her Majesty's Inspectorate of Prisons and Care Quality Commission (2018a). *Care for Elderly Prisoners Is Inconsistent and the Lack of Planning for An Ageing Population Is a Serious Defect, Say Inspectors.* Available from: www.justiceinspectorates.gov.uk/hmiprisons/media/press-releases/2018/10/care-for-elderly-prisoners-is-inconsistent-and-the-lack-of-planning-for-an-ageing-population-is-a-serious-defect-say-inspectors/ [Accessed on: 16 March 2020].

Her Majesty's Inspectorate of Prison and Care Quality Commission (2018b). *Social Care in Prisons in England and Wales: A Thematic Report.* Available from: www.justiceinspectorates.gov.uk/hmiprisons/wp-content/uploads/sites/4/2018/10/Social-care-thematic-2018-web.pdf [Accessed on: 16 March 2020].

Her Majesty's Prison and Probation Service (2018). *Model for Operational Delivery: Older Prisoners.* Available from: www.dementiaaction.org.uk/assets/0004/2423/MOD-for-older-prisoners__2_.pdf [Accessed on: 26 March 2020].

House of Commons Justice Committee (2013). *Older Prisoners: Fifth Report of Session 2013–14.* Available from: www.parliament.uk/documents/commons-committees/Justice/Older-prisoners.pdf [Accessed on: 16 March 2020].

House of Lords (2017a). Written question HL2097, 27 October.

House of Lords (2017b). Written question HL3278, 5 January.

The Howard League for Penal Reform (2016). *Indeterminate Sentences for Public Protection, Prison Information Bulletin.* Available from: https://howardleague.org/wp-content/uploads/2016/05/IPP-report.pdf [Accessed on: 23 March 2020].

Human Rights Watch (2012). *Old Behind Bars: The Aging Prison Population in the United States.* Available from: www.hrw.org/report/2012/01/27/old-behind-bars/aging-prison-population-united-states [Accessed on: 23 March 2020].

Independent Monitoring Board (2017). *Growing Old in Prison.* Available from: www.imb.org.uk/growing-old-prison/ [Accessed on: 20 March 2020].

Johnstone, T. (2019). *Ageing Prisoners Are Challenging the System Inside and Out.* Available from: www.agedcareinsite.com.au/2019/04/ageing-prisoners-are-challenging-the-system-inside-and-out/ [Accessed on: 16 March 2020].

Joyce, J., Maschi, T. (2016). *"In Here Time Stands Still": The Rights, Needs and Experiences of Older People in Prison.* Dublin: Irish Penal Reform Trust. Available from: www.iprt.ie/files/IPRT-Older_People_in_Prison_Report_web.pdf [Accessed on: 16 March 2020].

Kempker, E. (2003). Graying of American prisons: addressing the continued increase in geriatric inmates. *Corrections Compendium*, 28(6): 1–2.

Kerbs, J., Jolley, J. (2009). A commentary on age segregation for older prisoners: philosophical and pragmatic considerations for correctional systems. *Criminal Justice Review*, 34(1): 119–139.

Kim, K., Peterson, B, (2014). *Aging Behind Bars: Trends and Implications of Graying Prisoners in the Federal Prison System.* Washington, DC: Urban Institute.

Lammy, D. (2017). *The Lammy Review: An Independent Review into the Treatment of, and Outcomes for, Black, Asian and Minority Ethnic Individuals in the Criminal Justice System.* Available from: https://assets.publishing.service.gov.uk/government/uploads/system/uploads/attachment_data/file/643001/l ammy-review-final-report.pdf [Accessed on: 27 March 2020].

Law Council of Australia (2014). *Policy Discussion Paper on Mandatory Sentencing*, May. Available from: www.lawcouncil.asn.au/docs/ff85f3e2-ae36-e711-93fb-005056be13b5/1405-Discussion-Paper-Mandatory-Sentencing-Discussion-Paper.pdf [Accessed on: 25 March 2020].

Leigey, M.E., Schartmueller, D. (2019). The fiscal and human costs of life without parole. *The Prison Journal*, 99(2): 241–262.

Leigh, A. (2019). *The Second Convict Age: Explaining the Return of Mass Imprisonment in Australia*. Available from: http://andrewleigh.org/pdf/SecondConvictAge.pdf [Accessed on: 16 March 2020].

Mackay, A. (2015). Overcrowding in Australian prisons: the human rights implications. *Precedent*, 37(128): 37–41.

Mahoney, F.I., Barthel, D. (1965). Functional evaluation: the Barthel Index. *Maryland State Medical Journal*, 14: 56–61.

Mann, N. (2012). Ageing child sex offenders in prison: Denial, manipulation and community. *Howard Journal of Criminal Justice*, 51(4): 345–358.

McKillop, M., Boucher, A. (2018). *Aging Prison Populations Drive Up Costs: Older Individuals Have More Chronic Illnesses and Other Ailments That Necessitate Greater Spending*. Available from: www.pewtrusts.org/en/research-and-analysis/articles/2018/02/20/aging-prison-populations-drive-up-costs [Accessed on: 16 March 2020].

Medina, L., Sabo, S., Vespa, J. (2020). *Living Longer: Historical and Projected Life Expectancy in the United States, 1960 to 2060: Population Estimates and Projections*. Available from: www.census.gov/content/dam/Census/library/publications/2020/demo/p25-1145.pdf [Accessed on: 19 March 2020].

Ministry of Justice (2017). *Further Breakdown of the Prison Population by Age and Offence Group as at 31 December 2016*. London: Ministry of Justice.

Ministry of Justice (2018). *Prison Populations 2018 to 2023, England and Wales*. London: Ministry of Justice.

Ministry of Justice (2019a). *Prison Population Projections 2019 to 2024, England and Wales*. London: Ministry of Justice.

Ministry of Justice (2019b). *Offender Management Statistics Quarterly: April to June 2019*. London: Ministry of Justice.

Ministry of Justice (2019c). *Offender Management Statistics, Prison Population 2019*. London: Ministry of Justice.

Ministry of Justice, HM Prison Service and Her Majesty's Prison and Probation Service (2020). *Official Statistics: Prison Population Figures: 2020*. Available from: www.gov.uk/government/statistics/prison-population-figures-2020 [Accessed on: 16 March 2020].

Morris, N. (1974). *The Future of Imprisonment*. Chicago: University of Chicago Press.

Murphy, J. (1973). Marxism and retribution. *Philosophy and Public Affairs*, 2(3): 217–243.

National Offender Management Service (2015). *Prison Service Instruction: Adult Social Care 15/2015*.

National Research Council (2014). *The Growth of Incarceration in the United States: Exploring Causes and Consequences*. Washington, DC: The National Academies Press.

Nelson, B. (1992). The Minnesota sentencing guidelines: the effects of determinate sentencing on disparities in sentencing decisions. *Law & Inequality*, 10(2): 217–251.

Newburn, T. (2007). Tough on crime: penal policy in England and Wales. *Crime and Justice*, 36(1): 425–470.

Non, A.L., Román, J.C., Gross, C.L., Gilman, S.E., Loucks, E.B., Buka, S.L., Kubzansky, L.D. (2016). Early childhood social disadvantage is associated with poor health behaviours in adulthood. *Annals of Human Biology*, 43(2): 144–153.

Nowotny, K.M., Masters, R.K., Boardmen, J.D. (2016). The relationship between education and health among incarcerated men and women in the United States. *BMC Public Health*, 16: 916.

Office for National Statistics (2017). *National Population Projections: 2016-Based*. Available from: www.ons.gov.uk/releases/nationalpopulationprojections2016basedstatisticalbulletin [Accessed on: 19 March 2020].

Office for National Statistics (2018). *Living Longer – Office for National Statistics*. Available from: www.ons.gov.uk/peoplepopulationandcommunity/birthsdeathsandmarriages/ageing/articles/livinglongerhowourpopulationischangingandwhyitmatters/2018–08–13 [Accessed on: 19 March 2020].

O'Hara, K., Forsyth, K., Webb, R., Senior, J., Hayes, A.J., Challis, D., Fazel, S., Shaw, J. (2016). Links between depressive symptoms and unmet health and social care needs among older prisoners. *Age and Ageing*, 45: 158–163.

Olding, R. (2016). Call for complete rethink as prison population, recidivism explode. *The Sydney Morning Herald*, February 19. Available from: www.smh.com.au/national/nsw/recidivism-20160218-gmxmog.html [Accessed on: 25 March 2020].

Omolade, S. (2014). *The Needs and Characteristics of Older Prisoners. Results from the Surveying Prisoner Crime Reduction Survey*. London: Ministry of Justice.

The Osborne Association (2018). *The High Costs of Low Risk: The Crisis of America's Aging Prison Population*. Available from: www.osborneny.org/resources/the-high-costs-of-low-risk/the-high-cost-of-low-risk/ [Accessed on: 16 March 2020].

Opitz-Welke, A., Konrad, N., Welke, J., Bennefeld-Kersten, K., Gauger, V., Voulgaris, A. (2019). Suicide in older prisoners in Germany. *Frontiers in Psychiatry*, 10: 154.

Potter, E., Cashin, A., Chenoweth, L, Jeon, Y.-H. (2007). The healthcare of older inmates in the correctional setting. *International Journal of Prisoner Health*, 3(3): 204–213.

Prison Reform Trust (2019). *Bromley Briefings Prison Fact File: Winter 2019*. Available from: www.prisonreformtrust.org.uk/portals/0/documents/bromley%20briefings/Winter%20 2019%20Factfile%20web.pdf [Accessed on: 23 March 2020].

Public Health England (2017). *Health and Social Care Needs Assessments of the Older Prison Population. A Guidance Document*. London: Public Health England.

Sabol, W.J., Rosich, K., Kane, K.M., Kirk, D., Dubin, G. (2002). *Influences of Truth-in-Sentencing Reforms on Changes in States' Sentencing Practices and Prison Populations*. Washington, DC: Urban Institute.

Sawyer, W., Wagner, P. (2019). *Mass Incarceration: The Whole Pie 2019*. Available from: www.prisonpolicy.org/reports/pie2019.html [Accessed on: 16 March 2020].

Schnittker, J., Massoglia, M., Uggen, C. (2012). Out and down: incarceration and psychiatric disorders. *Prison and Men's Health*, 53(4): 448–464.

Senate Legal and Constitutional Affairs Committee (2013). *Legal and Constitutional Affairs References Committee Value of a Justice Reinvestment Approach to Criminal Justice in Australia*. Canberra: Senate Legal and Constitutional Affairs Committee Secretariat.

Senior, P., Forsyth, K., Walsh, E., O'Hara, K., Stevenson, C., Hayes, A., et al. (2013). Health and social care services for older male adults in prison: the identification of current service provision and piloting of an assessment and care planning model. *Health Services and Delivery Research*, 1(5).

Sentencing Council (2018). *Failure to Surrender to Bail, Bail Act 1976*, s.6. Available from: www.sentencingcouncil.org.uk/offences/magistrates-court/item/failure-to-surrender-to-bail/ [Accessed on: 23 March 2020].

The Sentencing Project (2017). *Still Life: America's Increasing Use of Life and Long-Term Sentences*. Available from: www.sentencingproject.org/wp-content/uploads/2017/05/Still-Life.pdf [Accessed on: 23 March 2020].

Shahani, A. (2017). The time does not fit the crime: eliminating mandatory minimums for nonviolent drug offenders in favor of judicial discretion. *Southwestern Journal of International Law*, 23: 445–467.

Sharupski, K.A., Gross, A., Schrack, J.A., Deal, J.A., Eber, G.B. (2018). The health of America's aging prison population. *Epidemiologic Reviews*, 40(1): 157–165.

Stemen, D., Rengifo, A., Wilson, J. (2006). *Of Fragmentation and Ferment: The Impact of State Sentencing Policies on Incarceration Rates, 1975–2002. Final Report to the National Institute of Justice*. Washington, DC: National Institute of Justice.

Stojkovic, S. (2007). Elderly prisoners: a growing and forgotten group within correctional systems vulnerable to elder abuse. *Journal of Elder Abuse and Neglect*, 19(3): 97–117.

Tonry, M. (2013). Sentencing in America, 1975–2025. *Crime and Justice*, 42(1): 141–198.

Trotter, C., Baidawi, S. (2015). Older prisoners: challenges for inmates and prison management. *Australian & New Zealand Journal of Criminology*, 200: 201.

Tucker, S., Hargreaves, C., Roberts, A., Anderson, I., Shaw, J., Challis, D. (2017). Social care in prison: emerging practice arrangements consequent upon the introduction of the 2014 care act. *The British Journal of Social Work*, 48(6): 1627–1644.

United Nations (2017). *World Population Prospects: The 2017 Revision*. Available from: https://population.un.org/wpp/Publications/Files/WPP2017_KeyFindings.pdf [Accessed on: 19 March 2020].

United States Sentencing Commission (2017). *Overview of Mandatory Minimum Penalties in the Federal Criminal Justice System*. Available from: www.ussc.gov/sites/default/files/pdf/research-and-publications/research-publications/2017/20170711_Mand-Min.pdf [Accessed on: 24 March 2020].

Visher, C., La Vigne, N., Travis, J. (2004). *Returning Home: Understanding the Challenges of Prisoner Reentry, Maryland Pilot Study: Findings from Baltimore*. Washington, DC: Urban Institute.

Von Hirsch, A. (1976). *Doing Justice*. New York: Hill & Wang.

Wangmo, T., Meyer, A.H., Bretschneider, W., Handtke, V., Kressing, R.W., Gravier, B., Bula, C., Elger, B.S. (2015). Ageing prisoners' disease burden: is being old a better predictor than time served in prison? *Gerontology*, 61: 116–123.

Wilkstrom, P.O.H., Treiber, K. (2016). Social disadvantage and crime: a criminological puzzle. *The American Behavioural Scientist*, 60(10): 1232–1259.

Williams, B.A., Stern, M.F., Mellow, J., Safer, M., Greifinger, R.B. (2012). Ageing in correctional custody: setting a policy agenda for older prisoner health care. *American Journal of Public Health*, 102(8): 1475–1481.

Williams, J.L. (2006). The aging inmate population: Southern states outlook. *Southern Legislative Conference*. Available from: www.slcatlanta.org/Publications/HSPS/aging_inmates_2006_lo.pdf [Accessed on: 26 March 2020].

World Health Organization (2018). *Ageing and Health*. Available from: www.who.int/newsroom/fact-sheets/detail/ageing-and-health [Accessed on: 19 March 2020].

World Health Organization and US National Institute of Aging (2011). *Global Health and Ageing*. Available from: www.who.int/ageing/publications/global_health.pdf?ua=1 [Accessed on: 19 March 2020].

World Prison Brief and Institute for Crime and Justice Policy Research (2019). *United Kingdom: England & Wales*. Available from: www.prisonstudies.org/country/united-kingdom-england-wales [Accessed on: 16 March 2020].

Yorston, G.A. (2015). *Managing Aggression and Violence in Older People*. London: The Royal College of Psychiatrists.

Yorston, G.A., Taylor, P.J. (2006). Commentary: older offenders – no place to go? *Journal of the American Academy of Psychiatry and the Law*, 34(3): 333–337.

2 Healthcare provision in prison

Joanne Brooke

Healthcare in prison

This section will explore the principles identified by the World Health Organization (Europe) of healthcare in prison (2014). It will then focus on countries within Europe, examining different approaches of providing healthcare, such as health authorities providing healthcare services within a prison, which is the approach in Norway, or the provision of healthcare services by the Ministry of Justice, which is the approach in France. Finally, an international perspective will include healthcare provision in Australian prisons. A number of frameworks and principles have informed their complex system of healthcare delivery, where state and tertiary governments are responsible and services commissioned and delivered vary among jurisdictions.

Principles of healthcare in prison

The World Health Organization (2014) have highlighted essential principles of healthcare in prison, and these elements are going to be introduced before addressing the implementation of different healthcare systems. The following 12 principles are discussed, recognising both human rights of prisoners (see Chapter 5) and the provision of ethical healthcare in prison (see Chapter 6):

1 Healthcare in prison is the responsibility of the state. This includes a duty of care for all people who are incarcerated. Duty of care requires the state to ensure the safety of prisoners and also ensure that their basic needs and human rights are met, which includes their right to healthcare.
2 The state must provide primary healthcare for prisoners, with appropriate staff, resources and facilities which are comparable to the standard of primary healthcare available in the community. The comparability of the provision of primary care in the prison and community is to ensure prisoners' care is equivalent to that of the community.
3 Healthcare professionals providing primary care for prisoners should preferably be employed independently of the prison administration, to

empower them to work within their professional codes of conduct, which needs to be both understood and accepted by the prison administration.

4   Healthcare professionals working in a prison setting must accept the prisoners they treat and care as patients, and as such are entitled to the same duty of care as patients they treat and care in the community.

5   A prisoner who is a patient has the right for healthcare professionals to respect and maintain their right to confidentiality, and care and treatment can only occur when the patient has provided informed consent.

6   The initial health screening and evaluation of prisoners on entering the prison system needs to be recognised as important and the best possible services should be provided to ensure a full and comprehensive screen and evaluation. Prison and healthcare professionals involved in this process must also acknowledge the need to refer prisoners to other institutions or specialist facilities as required.

7   A crucial element of prison healthcare is the continuity of care, especially when prisoners are transferred to another prison or released. It is the responsibility of the prison administration to organise and ensure continuity of care.

8   Prison administration are responsible for ensuring the environment of the prison does not expose the prisoner to any hazards likely to negatively affect their health.

9   The health of prisoners needs to be addressed more comprehensively than just by healthcare professionals, and prison staff should receive training in relevant healthcare issues to enable them to support the healthcare of prisoners.

10   The health inequalities of prisoners can be successfully addressed to support resettlement on release through the development of health resilience during their sentence, and this should be the aim of prison healthcare services.

11   All prison health services should aim to improve public health within the prison, supporting where possible the work of the prison to enable changes in attitudes and behaviours of prisoners.

12   Prison health services cannot work in isolation to achieve all of the previously mentioned principles and therefore need to be aligned and integrated into both regional and national health systems.

A European perspective of healthcare in prison

The Council of Europe Committee of Ministers adopted the European Prison Rules in 2006, and these have been amended and adopted again in 2019. Part III of the European Prison Rules provides regulation on healthcare, which overlaps with the essential principles identified by the WHO (2014), including elements of the organisation of healthcare in prison, medical and healthcare personnel, duties of medical practitioners and the provision of physical and mental healthcare. The rules regarding organisation of healthcare emphasise the need for the provision of healthcare to be integrated into and made comparable and compatible with regional and national health services of the country, and the importance of recognising that prisoners must not be discriminated against because of their legal situation. An aim of prison healthcare is to actively identify and treat both physical and mental health illnesses and provide access to specialist services in the community. The rules regarding medical and healthcare personnel state that every prison shall have at least one qualified general practitioner, who is available without delay in an emergency, and access to a qualified dentist and optician. The rules are more specific regarding the duties of medical practitioners, which include those emphasised by the principles of WHO (2014), but also more detailed elements of their role, some of which are expected from medical practitioners in any environment and some of which are specific to the prison environment, including:

- Medical practitioners and other healthcare professionals are responsible for maintaining patient (prisoner) confidentiality regarding health assessments, diagnosis and treatment.
- Medical practitioners and other healthcare professionals are responsible for diagnosing both physical and mental illness, providing appropriate treatment and ensuring the continuation of existing medical treatment.
- If there are any signs or indications a patient has been violently treated, medical practitioners and other healthcare professionals must record and the report this information to relevant prison administration.
- Medical practitioners and other healthcare professionals are responsible for supporting patients who have withdrawal symptoms resulting from illegal drug, medical or alcohol use.
- Medical practitioners and other healthcare professionals are responsible for identifying stress or other negative impacts on patients' psychological health due to deprivation of their liberty.
- Medical practitioners and other healthcare professionals are responsible for isolating patients who are suspected of an infectious illness for an appropriate period of time and providing the appropriate treatment.
- Medical practitioners and other healthcare professionals are responsible for ensuring patients with HIV are not isolated due to their HIV status.
- Medical practitioners and other healthcare professionals are responsible for identifying physical or psychological limitations of prisoners that may affect their resettlement after release.
- Medical practitioners and other healthcare professionals are responsible for assessing and identifying the level of fitness of each patient to engage in work and exercise.
- Medical practitioners and other healthcare professionals are responsible for organising the continuation of medical and psychiatric treatment on transfer to another prison or on release, engaging with community agencies with the patient's consent.

- Medical practitioners and other healthcare professionals are responsible for prisoners held under conditions of solitary confinement, visiting them daily and providing prompt medical care and treatment.
- Medical practitioners and other healthcare professionals report directly to the governor when a prisoner's physical or mental health is at a serious risk due to imprisonment or any condition of imprisonment, including solitary confinement.
- Furthermore, the medical practitioner is to advise on the provision of food and water; cleanliness of the prison and hygiene of the prisoners; sanitation, heating, lighting and ventilation of the prison; and the suitability of bedding provided.

Organisation of healthcare services in Europe

In many countries in Europe, the responsibility of providing healthcare within prisons has transferred from the prison administration to state health services. In France, this occurred in 1994, when prison healthcare provision became the responsibility of the General Health Directorate for Public Health Issues within the Ministry of Health. Whilst in England and Wales Prison Service, the responsibility for prison health was transferred to the National Health Service (NHS) in 2002 (WHO Europe, 2014); move information is provided on this later in this chapter. However, in Norway the provision of prison healthcare was transferred from the Ministry of Justice and became an integral part of the national public health service under the Ministry of Health and Care Services in 1988 (Nesset et al., 2011). Norway consists of four state-owned health authorities, and the aim of transferring the provision to the Ministry of Health and Care Services was to ensure comparable healthcare provision for prisoners as the general population. The expenses for the provision of prison healthcare is provided by the state but is organised by the municipal and county health administration where the prison is situated. Finally, large prisons in Norway have full healthcare services within the prison, although smaller prisons only have partial services (Nesset et al., 2011).

An international perspective of healthcare in prison – Australia

The Standards for health services in Australian prisons 1st edition (Royal Australian College of General Practitioners [RACGP], 2011) provides guidance and principles similar to the WHO Europe (2014) principles in healthcare in prison and the European Prison Rules (Council of Europe Committee of Ministers, 2006, 2019). The RACGP Standards highlights the unique challenges of providing healthcare for patients within a prison setting, as prison magnifies their clinical risks. Therefore, there is a need for healthcare professionals to be 'extra vigilant' to certain standards to provide safe and gold standard care to patients in prison. These standards include the need to support patients to make informed healthcare decisions; provision of interpreter services; clinical autonomy for all healthcare professionals; the development and continuity of a therapeutic relationship; the provision of respectful and culturally appropriate care; maintaining the privacy and confidentiality of patients health information; and the importance of engaging with outside services and the transfer of relevant health information.

In Australia, state and territory governments are both responsible for the provision of healthcare for prisoners. However, it varies by state (New South Wales, Victoria, Queensland, Western Australia, South Australia and Tasmania) and territory (of which there are three internal and seven external to mainland Australia, although not all are inhabited). However, most jurisdictions have a combination of services provided by the local Department of Health and the Department of Justice or Corrections, and therefore there is a combination of directly provided services, community services, or services provided by contracted external providers. The different models of healthcare for prisoners have been developed. For example in South Australia, primary care is provided within the prison setting, whereas secondary and tertiary healthcare is provided by the local public health system. In New South Wales and Victoria, primary, secondary and some tertiary services are available within the prison setting. However, the legislation and frameworks of the provision of healthcare for prisons as described by the RACGP (2011) is obligatory for all.

In Australia, primary healthcare is provided in each prison, and most prisons work closely with community-based primary health services, which also support the provision of healthcare for prisoners. In some prisons which are geographically isolated, in-reach services may be provided by community-based primary health services, such as care provided by general practitioners, although primary healthcare in prisons tends to be delivered by nurses. An element that differentiates community-based primary healthcare and prison primary healthcare is the focus of GP-led care in the community and nurse-led services in prison settings. Nurse-led services include initial assessment in reception, provision of medication and vaccinations. Most prisons also provide some secondary healthcare, which is the provision of specialist care, following a referral from a primary healthcare provider. Whereas, tertiary healthcare is specialist healthcare such as cancer management, and all jurisdictions provide access to some secondary and tertiary healthcare in the community, including general hospital inpatient care and emergency care. Alongside physical healthcare, all jurisdictions provide access to specialist mental healthcare, which is delivered in collaboration with local community mental health services; inpatient involuntary care is provided outside of the prison system (Australian Bulletin 123, 2014).

More recently, healthcare provision in Australian prisons has begun to focus on prisoners who are Aboriginal and Torres Strait Islander Australians, because of their poor health compared to non-indigenous Australians and because of the overrepresentation of these populations within Australian prisons, as they account for 28 per cent of the prison population, but only 3 per cent of the Australian population (Australian Bureau of Statistics, 2019). For example

Aboriginal and Torres Strait Islander Australians have a slightly lower age-standardised incidence rate for all cancers, but a significantly higher mortality rate compared to non-indigenous Australians (Australian Institute of Health and Welfare and Cancer Australia, 2013). Although there are many reasons for this, such as the types of cancer and the stage of diagnosis, healthcare within a prison setting needs to acknowledge and provide services to address this disparity.

Therefore, the provision of equitable healthcare for Aboriginal and Torres Strait Islander Australians is not the provision of equal treatment, but identifying their needs to support equal health outcomes, with the inclusion of culturally appropriate and safe healthcare in prison and continuation in the community (Kendall et al., 2020). This issue has been addressed by individual states; for example the South Australian Prison Services has identified, described and implemented a Model of Care for Aboriginal Prisoner Health (Sivak et al., 2017). The model of care identifies the chronic diseases that significantly affect this population, including communicable diseases and disabilities, and priority Aboriginal and Torres Strait Islander Australians health needs, within a holistic patient-centred approach. Further elements of the model include understanding the cultural and spiritual identity of the individual, improved communication and continuity of care as well as involvement of family members, flexible pathways, recovery and rehabilitation and linking individuals to community services prior to release (Sivak et al., 2017).

Healthcare provision in prisons in England

In England, since April 2013 the commissioning and provision of physical and mental health services for prisoners is the responsibility of NHS England, apart from drug and alcohol services. NHS England formed a tripartite collaborative to support this responsibility, which included Her Majesty's Prison and Probation Service (HMPPS) and Public Health England (PHE). More recently, this tripartite collaboration has expanded to include the Ministry of Justice and Department of Health and Social Care. This section will provide a brief history of the development of prison health in England. It will then discuss the three core objects to support the improvement of the health of prisoners, followed by ten key priorities from the current National Partnership Agreement for Prison Health 2018–2021. Finally, it will discuss current hospital use by prisoners and provide an example of primary care and mental healthcare within a prison setting.

Development of prison healthcare in England

Her Majesty's Chief Inspector for Health Care in Prisons (1996), an independent authority, published a highly critical document of the state of prison healthcare in England and Wales, which led to the formation of a Joint Prison Service and National Health Services Executive Working Group in 1999. The then newly formed working group identified a number of issues with the Prison

Service provision of healthcare for prisoners. These included multiple models of healthcare within English prisons, no strategic planning and development of healthcare provision, no clear lines of accountability, tensions between custody and care providers, different levels of integration to NHS care and a focus on treatment of illness rather than promoting health through processes rather than outcomes. Good practice was identified but occurred only because of dominant and passionate key leaders; otherwise healthcare staff lacked supervision, training and continuing development. The recommendation from this working group included the need for NHS health authorities and prisons to be jointly responsible for the healthcare of prisoners, and the development of a local prison health improvement strategy, which included both the provision of primary healthcare within prisons through internal and external resources, and secondary care within NHS hospitals either through outpatient clinics or as inpatients. The Department of Health became solely responsible for health policy in prisons in 2000 (Hayton and Boyington, 2006).

The Department of Health (2001) published their first health policy for prisons in England and Wales in 2001, which changed the approach to mental healthcare for prisoners with the introduction of in-reach services. In 2003, the Department of Health became responsible for the funding of primary care health provision in public prisons in England. The changes to the provision and responsibility of prison healthcare required the development of the National Partnership Agreement on the Transfer of Responsibility for Prison Health from the Home Office to the Department of Health in 2003 (NOMS, PHE and NHS England, 2013). This is an important event, which became the basis for change through a number of Prison Service Instructions (PSIs). Full commissioning responsibility for resources to provide prison health occurred in 2006, and Primary Care Trusts (PCTs) with their local prisons (excluding private prisons) created Prison Partnership Boards to identify and commission local services to address the needs of individual prisons within national agreements. In 2006 and 2007, a number of services were reformed, such as the implementation of an Integrated Drug Treatment System, and PCTs became responsible for Escort and Bedwatch services. These changes led to the second edition of the National Partnership Agreement between the Department of Health and Her Majesty's Prison Service for Accountability and Commissioning of Health Services for Prisoners in 2007 (NOMS, PHE and NHS England, 2013).

During this time and these changes, the responsibility of the Prison and Probation Services has transferred from the Home Office to the Ministry of Justice in 2007, and then to the National Offender Management Service (NOMS) in 2008, which has now changed to Her Majesty's Prison and Probation Service (HMPPS) in 2017. The responsibility of healthcare commissioning also changed in 2013 from PCTs, which ceased to exist, to Clinical Commissioning Groups (CCGs). However, in 2011 the Department of Health and the then-Ministry of Justice co-commissioned a programme to support, manage and treat the psychological health of prisoners with severe personality disorders, who were ultimately a serious harm to themselves and possibly others, through a reorganisation of the current Dangerous and Severe Personality Disorder Programme. Another reorganisation of care services from the then-NOMS to the Department of Health in 2011 included the responsibility for commissioning non-clinical substance misuse services, which completed the transfer of all prison healthcare to NHS Trusts, with the exception of healthcare within private prisons.

The National Partnership Agreement was updated again by NHS England in 2013 to recognise the need for the tripartite agreement of NHS England, NOMS and Public Health England (PHE) to develop priorities, commission and deliver healthcare in prisons in England. The responsibilities of each governing body are clearly outlined: NHS England is responsible for the delivery of all healthcare, NOMS for the provision of prisons and prisoners' daily life including occupational rehabilitation, whilst PHE provided expert public health guidance and tools to both NOMS and NHS England, but were not directly responsible for commissioning or managing prisons or healthcare services. In 2016, PHE completed and published the Rapid Review of evidence of the impact of health outcomes of NHS-commissioned health services for people in secured and detained settings to inform future priorities and health interventions (PHE, 2016). The Rapid Review identified both areas of strength and areas for further improvements, including developing a whole prison approach, data and intelligence, community engagement, and more relevant to this chapter, strategy, leadership and partnerships and frontline services which are described in more depth later.

The strengths of strategy, leadership and partnerships included the collaboration of NHS England, NOMS and PHE, due to the clear roles, responsibilities and accountabilities outlined in the National Partnership Agreement (2013). However, areas for further improvement included the need for transparent links with community healthcare provision and community safety partnerships. A further need identified was that of the development of population outcomes rather than individual outcomes to support a combined purpose within the partnerships and to bridge the gap between a focus on security versus a focus on health. The need also remained to enable commissioning to support acute and community care with effective pathways throughout prisoners' contact with the criminal justice system and return to the community.

PHE identified the vast improvement in frontline services in healthcare provision in prisons and the effectiveness of local services since 2006, when NHS England became responsible for commissioning. An important element highlighted was the employment of appropriately qualified healthcare professionals who were registered with relevant national professional bodies, which supported an improvement in both clinical standards and accountability. A further strength identified was the introduction and implementation of patient advice and liaison services (PALS), a process for complaints, which is the process embedded in NHS Trusts outside prison settings, alongside other mechanisms to obtain service user feedback, in this case, prisoners as patients. Finally, the implementation of national standards, such as those by the National Institute for Health and Care Excellence (NICE), was found to support the clinical improvement of the delivery of services. However, areas for further improvement included elements on cost effectiveness, alongside the need for further education for healthcare professionals regarding prison health, prison staff and healthcare professionals working collaboratively to support understanding of each other's role and prisoner's health, sharing good local practice at a national level and further engagement with Health Education England.

National Partnership Agreement for Prison Healthcare in England 2018–2021

More recently, the National Partnership Agreement of 2013 has been superseded by the National Partnership Agreement for Prison Healthcare in England 2018–2021 (HM Government, NHS England, 2018), with the inclusion of five partners: the Ministry of Justice, Her Majesty's Prison and Probation Service, Public Health England, the Department of Health and Social Care and NHS England. This collaboration has identified three core objectives: first, to improve the health and well-being of prisoners and reduce health inequalities between prisoners and those living in the community; second, to reduce reoffending through increasing support and rehabilitation by directly addressing drivers of offending that are health-related; and third, to support the continuity of access and care through the prison setting, pre-custody and post-custody in the community. The five partners of this agreement aim to address these three core overarching objectives by focusing on the following ten key priorities:

1 An emphasis on collaborative working across all sections of prison and health and social care, through the provision of multi-agency approaches to improve practice and reduce the number of incidences of self-harm and suicide of adults in prison, whilst further embedding shared learning (addresses the first and third core objectives).
2 The continuation and emphasis across the multi-agency approach to reduce the impact of substance misuse, whilst simultaneously addressing the negative risks associated with misuse and possible harms to enable the right support, help and treatment at the right time (addresses all three core objectives).
3 The need for collaboration to support and improve the mental health and well-being of prisoners, which will include timely and appropriate assessments, treatment and continuation of care through informed transfers, with a particular focus on the mental health needs of prisoners with protected characteristics (addresses all three core objectives).
4 A focus on supporting older prisoners and those with serious illnesses through ensuring the continuation of improvements to health and social care, with an emphasis on prevention, diagnosis, treatment and end-of-life care. Alongside the implementation of evidence-based care which

addresses both the needs of the population and of individual prisoners (addresses the first and third core objectives).

5   The improvement of data and intelligence collection, including the quality of the data and the ability to share the data between collaborative part- ners. This priority includes data sharing throughout the offenders' jour- nal through the criminal justice system, to enable continuity of care and inform the development of effective health outcome measures (addresses all three core objectives).

6   The five collaborators need to develop policy collectively to ensure pris- oners' health and social care needs are addressed throughout the criminal justice system through shared objectives, with the commitment to fairness, diversity and equality (addresses all three core objectives).

7   A focus on continuing to improve commissioning between health and justice partners, and their external links with local authorities, probation service and health commissioning in the community, to ensure continua- tion and consistency of care pre- and post-custody (addresses all three core objectives).

8   The development of a whole prison approach to address the health and well-being of prisoners, including prison regimes and activities, as well as staffing, which promotes an environment that reduces violence and is inclusive of those with protected characteristics (addresses all three objectives).

9   The improvement of prisoners' access to preventive, diagnostic and screen- ing programmes that are available for the general public, and the improve- ment of detection, surveillance and management of infectious diseases, alongside adequate data and intelligence collection to respond to and report outbreaks and incidents (addresses only the first objective).

10   Lastly, to ensure that all health and social care services are implemented in alignment with and to support current and future changes in prison estate design, infrastructure, function and operation (addresses all three objectives).

Prisoners' use of hospital services in England and Wales

All of the National Partnership Agreements for prison healthcare in England have concentrated on the progress and improvement of healthcare for prisoners, with a focus on primary health and mental health services, and an acknowl- edgement of the need for secondary healthcare to be linked with local NHS Trusts. However, a contemporary evaluation of the data reported in 'Locked out? Prisoners' use of hospital care', which analysed over 110,000 hospital med- ical records of prisoners from 112 prisons in England and Wales, across 2017 and 2018 (Davies et al., 2020) suggests prisoners are still not obtaining hospital care that is equitable to that of the general population. From the data, it was identified that prisoners had 24 per cent fewer hospital admissions and outpa- tient appointments than the general population when matched for age and sex demographics, and worryingly 40 per cent of outpatient appointments for prisoners were not attended. The process of outpatient appointments to occur via video or telephone has been developed, and 3 per cent of outpatient appointments for the general population occurs through this method. However, this is compared to only 2 per cent of outpatient appointments attended by prisoners, when this approach would appear to support attendance and reduce pressure on prison services to support transport and staff to escort prisoners.

The report also identified the reason for prisoners' use of hospital services, which was overwhelmingly due to external causes rather than a disease affecting their health; for example injury and poisoning accounted for 18 per cent of prisoners' admission to the hospital, which is compared to 6 per cent in the general adult population. Another example of prisoners' use of hospital services was due to external causes, such as head injuries, which accounted for 508 hospital admissions and a further 415 emergency department visits. The injuries recorded regarding head injuries included fractures of the skull and facial bones, intracranial injuries and open wounds. An element that has been identified and addressed but requires further action is more than 25 per cent of all inpatient admissions by prisoners were recorded to have psychoactive substance use (Davies et al., 2020). This data also suggests that prisoners with physical health needs and illnesses may not be attending routine outpatient appointments because of the considerable number of external trauma admissions by prisoners, as prisons have limited capacity to escort prisoners to hospital.

HMP Birmingham

This section provides an overview of an example of prison healthcare in an English prison, HMP Birmingham. This section is informed by information from a Health Needs Assessment (HNA) that occurred in 2015 (Offenders Health Needs Assessment [OHNA], 2015). The HNA is a systematic method for identifying priorities and allocating resources to improve the health of the prison population (PHE, 2014). The general aim of an HNA in a prison setting is to improve the overall health and well-being of prisoners and to reduce the inequalities in prisoners' health and their access to healthcare compared to the general population. The development of an HNA toolkit for prescribed places of detention in England and Wales was developed by PHE, NHS England, NOMS, the Youth Justice Board and Public Health Wales. Prescribed places of detention are wider than just prisons and includes young offender institutions, secure training centres, secure children's homes and immigration removal centres.

HMP Birmingham is a Victorian prison opened in 1849, although the prison has been refurbished with the most extensive refurbishment occurring in 2004. The refurbishment included the building of a health centre, which includes inpatient care for prisoners with either physical or mental health needs, an education centre and workshops and a gym. Following this refurbishment, HMP Birmingham had 12 wings, with a capacity for 1,450. However, since a couple of incidents in 2016 and 2017, the capacity has been reduced to hold around 1,028 prisoners over 11 wings. The remaining wings are used to separate vulnerable prisoners, sex offenders, those going through detoxification and older prisoners, as well as including a first night centre. HMP Birmingham is a category B (prisoners who are a risk to the public but may not require maximum security, but for whom escape still needs to be made very difficult) and a category C prison (prisoners who cannot be trusted in open conditions but who are unlikely to try to escape). HMP Birmingham holds both sentenced and remand prisoners and was operated privately from 2011 to 2018. An important factor affecting this prison is the high turnover of prisoners, due to holding prisoners on remand and those completing short sentences (less than five years), which has been estimated to represent a population churn of 4.5 per year.

Primary healthcare

Primary Health Care in HMP Birmingham is provided by Birmingham Community Healthcare NHS Foundation Trust, which is led by a GP who is directly employed. The GP provision is comparable to that of a community GP practice; clinics are held within the prison Monday to Friday morning by two GPs with an average of 36 appointments each clinic, and afternoon clinics Monday to Thursday by one GP with an average of 14 appointments each clinic. This may reflect the waiting time for prisoners to see a GP which is on average between 6 and 15 days. A GP also covers the evening reception from 6 to 9 pm, to support the health assessment of new prisoners. Nurses also provide a number of clinics, which are delivered from both the health centre and different wings across the prison. These include general clinics, such as vaccinations, well-man and sexual health clinics and clinics for older prisoners, alongside specialist clinics focusing on specific diseases such as diabetes, COPD and wounds, and mental health clinics, all of which have a dedicated nurse specialising in this field. Other clinics include the provision of physiotherapy (twice a week), optician (once a week, and an extra clinic once a month for vulnerable prisoners), podiatry (twice a week) and dental clinics (nine times a week). However, during the OHNA (2015), the 'did not attend' rate by prisoners was 42 per cent, which had been recognised and plans implemented to reduce. Primary healthcare is supported by a 15-bedded inpatient ward staffed by the primary healthcare team.

Mental healthcare

Mental healthcare services at HMP Birmingham are provided by Birmingham and Solihull Mental Health Trust. The staff are permanently based at the prison and provide comprehensive services, including both primary and secondary mental health services as well as dual diagnosis and forensic mental health services, liaising extensively with both health and justice mental health services and other external agencies. On average, OHNA (2015) estimates 125 new mental health assessments are undertaken every month, and secondary care provided support for 112 patients (prisoners) every month on their 15-bedded mental health inpatient unit. The unit contains 15 individual cells, of which two are gated to provide constant observation. The unit admits patients for assessment and stabilisation, from both internally within the prison and externally from other prisons. Much like any inpatient setting, weekly ward rounds occur to review patient's progress and manage discharge. Two registered mental health nurses and three healthcare officers (prison staff) staff the ward daily; during the night, this decreases to one nurse and two healthcare officers. Therapeutic interventions occur daily, including a range of psychology and talking therapies, self-help strategies and engagement sessions.

Planned and unplanned secondary care

Planned secondary care has been a focus within the healthcare department of HMP Birmingham, with the allocation of five appointments per day per week – three in the morning and two in the afternoon – to escort patients to the hospital. However, the team identified that it is sometimes difficult to manage the caseload within the number of allocated appointments available because of the number of prisoners within HMP Birmingham (OHNA, 2015). A high number of visits involved patients needing an X-ray; therefore HMP Birmingham have begun to X-ray within the prison, which is supported by radiography staff from Birmingham City Hospital. Following the need for X-ray, a high number of visits were due to dialysis, ultrasound and fracture clinics or unplanned visits to the emergency department.

Challenges of providing healthcare in prison

This section will explore the challenges faced by healthcare professionals within a prison setting, with discussions regarding providing primary care, including healthcare to older prisoners and mental healthcare (Solell and Smith, 2019; Samele et al., 2016; Bedard et al., 2016). It will then focus on the challenges and barriers experienced by different healthcare professionals, such as nurses. Finally, it will discuss in depth one particular area which is prominent in the aging prison population, palliative care and the unique challenges of providing it in prison. A number of issues in the provision of healthcare have been highlighted such as communication with prison staff and the prisoner's family members, and prison restrictions, which prevent interventions to relieve pain and improve quality of life of the prisoner at the end of their life (Courtwright et al., 2008). These challenges have a practical and emotional impact on prison staff and healthcare professionals (Turner and Peacock, 2017).

Challenges of providing primary care

The challenges of providing primary care in the prison setting have been identified and include the health needs of this unique population, specifically the
need to address health promotion in areas such as smoking cessation, diet and
exercise, sexual health, substance misuse and communicable diseases, alongside
the need to manage long-term chronic diseases, such as respiratory conditions,
ischemic heart disease and cardiovascular risk factors, diabetes and epilepsy
(Condon et al., 2007).

Health promotion

An element of primary care provision is health promotion. Health professionals
working in a prison setting may find health promotion with prisoners challenging, such as advising prisoners regarding an appropriate amount of exercise
and the consumption of a healthy diet, as prisoners will ultimately have limited
ability to make autonomous decisions. Male prisoners have reported eating
less than three fruits and vegetables a day, although meals provided by the
prison support the eating of five fruits and vegetables daily (Lester et al., 2003).
Therefore, although healthy nutritious meals may appear on the menu, prisoners may not always view this as the case. Similarly, all prisons have regulations
on the time spent outside and exercising, elements of overcrowding and a lack
of prison staff may negatively affect the prison regime and prevent prisoners'
ability to exercise (Condon et al., 2007). Health promotion also includes sexual
health; within a male prison, this needs to be specifically addressed because of
the high incidence of sexually transmitted infections (STI), a lack of prisoners'
knowledge regarding STIs, and behaviour that leaves prisoners at risk of an STI
(Recio et al., 2016). Sexual health promotion alongside screening and treatment needs to be provided within primary care provision, although a reduction in STIs will require a prison-wide approach to education and changes to
prisoners' behaviours.

Chronic disease management

A challenge for primary care services within a prison setting and within a number of community settings is the provision of specialist care for chronic disease
management. Clinical nurse specialists or advance nurse practitioners are nurses
who possess specialist knowledge, skills, competencies and experience and who
are competent to work as an autonomous healthcare professional (Royal College of Nursing [RCN], (2009). The involvement of clinical nurse specialists
or advance nurse practitioners within patient care and treatment significantly
improves patient outcomes (RCN, 2009). However, within primary healthcare in a prison, this would require specialist nurses in respiratory, cardiovascular
disease, diabetes and epilepsy to support patients' needs; although a nurse may
specialise in one of these diseases, it is common practice for them to support

patients across the spectrum of diseases. Regarding challenges for the provision of care for individual diseases, in England and Wales, respiratory diseases have been supported by the ban on smoking tobacco within a prison. The challenges of managing diabetes in a prison setting are complex; there is a need for control of syringes and needles, which disempowers patients to manage their own diabetes, and prisoners rely on nurses working within the regime to manage their diabetes, which needs to be addressed prior to release (Reagan et al., 2016). Challenges across chronic disease management, but identified within the management of cardiovascular disease are the multiple correctional and medical notes, and the involvement of healthcare professionals in non-medical decisions, such as the need for a prisoner to have a bottom bunk or clearance for a certain job, which prevent the provision of person–centred healthcare (Thomas et al., 2016).

Challenges of providing mental healthcare

The challenges of mental health professionals providing in-reach services are complex; one element identified is the timely completion of new referrals whilst managing their current workload (Samele et al., 2016). Another challenge is understanding the mental health illnesses a patient may have previously had diagnosed; finding relevant information is sometimes difficult because of the lack of engagement before prison with mental health services, and a full assessment and re-diagnose often needs to occur (Samele et al., 2016). A common misperception by prisoners is they believe they have schizophrenia, when this is not always the case. A further challenge identified by mental healthcare professionals is the limited time patients were available to engage in therapeutic interventions because of the time they spent locked in their cells, which also restricted them to engage in healthy activities such as going to the gym or attending educational opportunities (OHNA, 2015).

Inpatient beds within prison or secure settings are always limited and may involve a patient being transferred to another prison for this level of care, which causes the patient distress. Nurses working in an inpatient ward encountered difficulties stemming from patients being admitted with challenging behaviours, which were not always related to mental health problems, but rather a consequence of their complex histories, including exposure to trauma throughout their life (Leidenfrost and Antonius, 2020). These patients tended to be transferred to mental health inpatients as prison staff could not manage their behaviours in the prison setting. Thus, the challenge of mental healthcare professionals was to work with patients with both mental health illnesses and disruptive behaviours due to their life history.

Challenges faced by nurses

Nurses face challenges when providing assessment, treatment and care in the prison settings, such as the need to negotiate boundaries and conflict between custody and caring (Weiskopf, 2005; Dhaliwal and Hirst, 2016), the need to create a caring environment in the prison setting (Weiskopf, 2005; Williams and Heavey, 2014), the need to remain vigilant around convicted offenders (Solell and Smith, 2019) and the attitude and language of correctional staff (Williams and Heavey, 2014; Solell and Smith, 2019).

Conflict between custody and care

The conflict between custody and care experienced by nurses providing care involves important elements that have been defined by Dhaliwal and Hirst (2016), including conflicting ethical and philosophical ideologies, correctional priorities overriding nursing priorities and the challenge of providing care but the need to maintain security. The conflict of ethical and philosophical ideologies may occur because of the unique setting of healthcare provision in a prison setting. Nurses may find the security boundaries imposed by prison authorities as challenging and a limitation to provide patient care to the best of their ability. Nurses need to negotiate the boundaries between the two cultures of caring for a patient and the responsibilities of the prison to ensure custody of the prisoner. Negotiating these boundaries creates complex challenges and frustrations for them as they identify the limits set by custodial staff (Weiskopf, 2005). Nurses have stated that they feel uncomfortable that the security of the prison is more important and prioritised over the care they need to provide to their patients (Solell and Smith, 2019). A boundary for nurses caring for patients in custody was the lack of ability to disclose any information about themselves or demonstrate empathy to patients through touch, which left nurses feeling regret that they had not cared for their patients to the best of their ability (Weiskopf, 2005).

The conflict nurses experience when providing care in the prison setting affects the quality of care they provide, and this is further influenced by the increased health needs of prisoners (White and Larsson, 2012). A challenge identified by nurses is the conundrum of whether to know a patient's criminal background, as this may be contrary to their own standards and beliefs, and nurses feared this may affect the care they provide (White and Larsson, 2012). However, nurses working in prison settings in the UK have recently described how some of the barriers between custody and care are beginning to change, with prison officers receiving training in healthcare, which supported collaborative working with a unified rather than opposing approach (Powell et al., 2010). Conflicts between the delivery of healthcare and the prison regime still remained, as providing services in the wider prison without the support of prison officers was time consuming and affected their role as healthcare professionals. For instance one nurse explained the provision of a vaccination clinic, where she was providing the vaccinations but also collecting the prisoners from their cell to bring them to the clinic (Powell et al., 2010).

Creating a caring environment in the prison setting

The prison environment must be recognised as affecting both nursing practice and nurses' ability to provide the same care when working in environments outside of the prison. Nurses can not ignore the stark and harsh nature of prison environments and the reality that patients were prisoners, who are there to be punished for the crimes they had committed (Weiskopf, 2005). A further problem identified by nurses was the influence of the prison environment on fellow nurses' attitudes towards the patients and the belief that some nurses did not like the patients they were caring for, which was believed to be 'a sad thing' (Weiskopf, 2005). Whereas, Solell and Smith (2019) identified two approaches nurses applied when caring for patients in the prison environment. First, there is a need to understand the complicated backgrounds of prisoners, whilst the nurses maintained their own caring values and compassion when providing care, regardless of the patients' background and the crimes they had committed. Second, nurses adopted a humanistic approach to the provision of the best care possible to prisoners as humans within the constraints of the prison.

Need to remain vigilant

The need for nurses to remain vigilant was beyond that of the need to understand the volatile environment of a prison setting; it was due to the belief that some prisoners tried to manipulate healthcare professionals for a secondary gain, such as acquiring medication, time out of their cell or just a social diversion (Weiskopf, 2005; Peternelji-Taylor, 2004). This challenge was addressed by nurses by being 'firm, fair and consistent', which was considered necessary to prevent prisoners from taking advantage of them for secondary gains, especially when prisoners exaggerated their symptoms or did not present their complaints honestly (White and Larsson, 2012; Weiskopf, 2005). The firm, fair and consistent approach developed by nurses was the development of an objective approach to care. This approach supported the collection of accurate assessment information and the development of a therapeutic relationship, which was suitable for the prison environment as supported nurses to provide appropriate treatment and maintain their professional role (Solell and Smith, 2019). However, it has also been recognised that there is a possibility that patients within the prison setting may not have the understanding or knowledge to present their symptoms in an informative way, and therefore nurses need the skills to assess patients to ensure accurate diagnosis and treatment (Williams and Heavey, 2014).

Attitude and language of correctional staff

The majority of prison protocols require correctional staff/prison officers to be present when nurses complete assessments and provide care and treatments to prisoners. Nurses working within these constraints have identified that prison officers' attitudes are a barrier to the provision of appropriate care. This is because prison officers are a constant reminder of the custodial setting and the power difference between the officer and prisoner, and within this context, it is a challenge for nurses to provide empathetic and compassionate care (Solell and Smith, 2019). This challenge was addressed through nurses involving prison officers as part of the multidisciplinary team, which helped them to understand the healthcare needs of the prisoners they were there to support (Powell et al., 2010). Nurses also identified the need but also the challenge of having to be part of both worlds, the need to be seen as a colleague by prison officers and the need to be trusted as a healthcare professional by prisoners, which was a constant balancing act for nurses (Weiskopf, 2005).

Challenges of providing palliative and end-of-life care

Providing palliative and end-of-life care for patients in the prison setting can be particularly challenging for healthcare professionals. In England and Wales, the older prison population is significantly increasing, as discussed in Chapter 1, and 50 per cent of deaths in custody are accounted for by older prisoners (Ministry of Justice, 2019). Hospice provision for prisoners has begun to be introduced in a number of prisons in England and Wales, although with a limited number of beds. An important distinction between palliative care and end-of-life care exists, although these terms are often used interchangeably. Palliative care encompasses end-of-life care, but it has a much wider scope and involves all care and treatment for an illness which has no cure, such as controlling symptoms and providing support with social, psychological and spiritual needs to maintain an optimal quality of life for the patient (Krau, 2016). End-of-life care is the end part of palliative care, when a patient is nearing the end of their life, which often encompasses their last six months. It focuses on supporting a patient to die with dignity; in the community this would be in the place of their choice (Krau, 2016). In the unique prison setting, patients do not have the choice to die at home amongst their family, placing more pressure on the provision of hospice care within prisons. Healthcare professionals identified the lack of choice prisoners have regarding their place of death, negatively affecting their own experience of providing end-of-life care for the prisoner (Panozzo et al., 2020).

Challenge of restraints

A challenge for all healthcare professionals which has been highlighted and repeatedly criticised by the Prison and Probation Ombudsman (PPO, 2013, 2017) is the 'practice of restraining ill or dying prisoners' and the need for risk assessments to ensure restraints are appropriate to risk posed by an unwell prisoner. The challenge for healthcare professionals is to provide end-of-life care when the patient is excessively restrained. This has been highlighted by the PPO since 2013, when a number of cases were reported, which included a prisoner remaining restrained although in a coma, a prisoner who died whilst still handcuffed to a prison officer. In the 16 cases examined, restraints were not removed until 24 hours or less before the prisoner died (PPO, 2013). There is a need to address and maintain the balance between security and humanity. The challenges for healthcare professionals in this very difficult situation include the provision of appropriate and timely medication for both pain and other symptoms (Turner et al., 2011; Turner and Peacock, 2017). However, prisoners receiving palliative care have identified and understood the support and confines of healthcare professionals because of the prison regime. One prisoner expressed,

> I don't think the staff don't care because, to be honest with you, I think the staff do care, a lot of them do care about you, but I think it's just there's no [pause] there's no system in place for anybody who is in real bad pain.
> (Turner and Peacock, 2017, p. 61)

Challenges of involving family

Healthcare professionals have discussed the challenges of caring for a patient who is dying, without their family members being present due to the restraints of the prison regime (Panozzo et al., 2020). Close family members and friends are an essential element to an individual's end-of-life care and a requirement to provide holistic care for the individual. Yet, this is often forgotten in the prison setting. Family members of patients being cared for in secure prison hospital wards still had their visits restricted, even when their relative was close to death. A further concern for all was bringing children into this environment to enable them to say goodbye to their relative, as this was not a supportive or appropriate environment (Panozzo et al., 2020).

In the UK, the Dying Well in Custody Charter (Ambitions for Palliative and End of Life Care Partnership, 2018) has been developed, which is a national framework for local action, alongside an assessment tool to support dying well in a prison setting. The charter contains six ambitions, which address some of the issues raised within this section on challenges: 1 each person is seen as an individual; 2 each person gets fair access to care; 3 comfort and well-being are maximised; 4 care is coordinated; 5 all staff are prepared to care; and 6 each community is prepared to help. With regard to the inclusion of family members of a prisoner who is receiving end-of-life care, the charter states that information and support will be provided to close family and friends, and their concerns listened to. A Family Liaison Officer will also be appointed to support the family, including access to be with their relative, unless otherwise indicated, and visits at the end of life, including out of hours regardless of the individual's location. However, the implementation of this charter has yet to be documented.

Emotional challenges

The emotional challenges of palliative care and end-of-life care affect healthcare professionals, prison staff and prisoners. Healthcare professionals' challenges described in this section can be viewed as constraints on how they provide care to terminally ill prisons, which evokes a philosophical tension between prison regimes and their founding principles of palliative care (Panozzo et al., 2020). Prisoner officers also find supporting prisoners at the end of life emotionally challenging as this is not an aspect of the job they considered when they decided to join the prison service. They have identified the need to find ways to cope with this emotional element of their work, especially as they recognised this was the first time many of them had come into contact with a person who was dying (Turner and Peacock, 2017). Fellow prisoners also experience the dying of a fellow prisoner as emotionally challenging. Prisoners who have been serving a long sentence and have fewer or no contacts with family members and friends, will have developed relationships with fellow prisoners, who will experience loss and require support (Turner and Peacock, 2017).

Summary

The World Health Organization has identified 12 essential principles of healthcare in prison, which recognise both human rights and ethical healthcare. In Europe, these principles have been further defined in the European Prison Rules, which provide guidance on the provision, implementation and delivery of healthcare in prison settings. The provision of healthcare in prisons has moved from being the responsibility of prison services to the responsibility of state health services. This change has occurred globally; in the Prison Service in England and Wales, this was fully realised in 2006. More recently, in England, healthcare in prison is guided by the National Partnership Agreement for Prison Healthcare 2018–2021. However, improvements in healthcare for prisoners is still required, as prisoners are still not accessing equivalent healthcare when compared to the general public. The final element of this chapter discusses the challenges of healthcare professionals and especially nurses in providing care to prisoners within the prison setting, and the negative impact of those challenges in creating a caring environment and providing end-of-life care.

References

Ambitions for Palliative and End of Life Care Partnership (2018). *Dying Well in Custody Charter Self-Assessment Tool. A National Framework for Local Action.* Available from: http://endoflifecareambitions.org.uk/wp-content/uploads/2018/06/Dying-Well-in-Custody-Self-Assessment-Tool-June-2018.pdf [Accessed on: 2 June 2020].

Australian Bureau of Statistics (2019). *Prisoners in Australia*, cat. no. 4517.0. Canberra: Australian Bureau of Statistics.

Australian Government (2014). *Bulletin 123: Prisoner Health Services in Australia.* Canberra, Australia: Australian Institute of Health and Welfare.

Australian Institute of Health and Welfare, & Cancer Australia (2013). *Cancer in Aboriginal and Torres Strait Islander People of Australia: An Overview.* Canberra, Australia: Australian Institute of Health and Welfare, & Cancer Australia.

Bedard, R., Metzger, L., Williams, B. (2016). Ageing prisoners: an introduction to geriatric health-care challenges in correctional facilities. *International Review of the Red Cross*, 98(3): 917–939.

Condon, L., Hek, G., Harris, F. (2007). A review of prison health and its implications for primary nursing in England and wales: the research evidence. *Journal of Clinical Nursing*, 16: 1201–1209.

Council of Europe Committee of Ministers (2006). *European Prison Rules*. Available from: https://rm.coe.int/european-prison-rules-978-92-871-5982-3/16806ab9ae#:~:text=40.3%20Prisoners%20shal l%20have%20access, from%20which%20prisoners%20may%20suffer [Accessed on: 2 June 2020].

Council of Europe Committee of Ministers (2019). *Revised Rules and Commentary to Recommendation CM/REC (2006)2 of the Committee of Ministers to Member States on the European Prison Rules*. Available from: https://rm.coe.int/pc-cp-2018-15-e-rev-3-epr-2006-with-changes-and-commentary-08–10–18/16808e4ac1 [Accessed on: 2 June 2020].

Courtwright, A., Raphael-Grimm, T., Collichio, F. (2008). Shackled: the challenge of caring for an incarcerated patient. *American Journal of Hospice and Palliative Medicine*, 25(4): 315–317.

Davies, M., Rolewicz, L., Schlepper, L., Fagunwa, F. (2020). *Research Report February 2020. Locked Out? Prisoners' Use of Hospital Care*. Available from: www.nuffieldtrust.org.uk/files/2020-02/prisoners-use-of-hospital-services-main-report.pdf [Accessed on: 2 June 2020].

Department of Health (2001). *Changing the Outlook*. Available from: https://webarchive.nationalarchives.gov.uk/20110504020501/www.dh.gov.uk/prod_consum_dh/groups/dh_digitalassets/@dh/@en/documents/digitalasset/dh_4034228.pdf [Accessed on: 2 June 2020].

Dhaliwal, K., Hirst, S. (2016). Caring in correctional nursing: a systematic search and narrative synthesis. *Journal of Forensic Nursing*, 12(1): 5–12.

Hayton, P., Boyington, J. (2006). Prisons and health reforms in England and Wales. *American Journal of Public Health*, 96(1): 1730–1733.

Her Majesty's Chief Inspector for Health Care in Prisons (1996). *Patient or Prisoner? A New Strategy for Health Care in Prisons*. Available from: www.justiceinspectorates.gov.uk/hmiprisons/wp-content/uploads/sites/4/2014/08/patient_or_prisoner_rps.pdf [Accessed on: 2 June 2020].

Her Majesty's Government, NHS England (2018). *National Partnership Agreement for Prison Healthcare in England 2018–2021*. Available from: https://assets.publishing.service.gov.uk/government/uploads/system/uploads/attachment_data/file/767832/6.4289_MoJ_National_health_partnership_A4-L_v10_web.pdf [Accessed on: 2 June 2020].

Kendall, S., Lighton, S., Sherwood, J., Baldry, E., Sullivan, E.A. (2020). Incarcerated aboriginal women's experiences of accessing healthcare and the limitations of the 'equal treatment' principle. *International Journal for Equity in Health*, 19: 48.

Krau, S. (2016). The difference between palliative care and end-of-life care: more than semantics. *Nursing Clinics of North America*, 5(3): ix–x.

Leidenfrost, C.M., Antonius, D. (2020). Incarceration and trauma: a challenge for the mental health care delivery system. *Assessing Trauma in Forensic Contexts*, 85–110.

Lester, C., Hamilton-Kirkwood, I., Jones, N. (2003). Health indicators in a prison population: asking prisoners. *Health Education Journal*, 62: 341–349.

Ministry of Justice (2019). *Safety in Custody Statistics, England and Wales: Deaths in Prison Custody to December 2018 and Self-harm to September 2018*. Available from: https://assets.publishing.service.gov.uk/government/uploads/system/uploads/attachment_data/file/774880/safety-in-custody-bulletin-2018-Q3.pdf [Accessed on: 2 June 2020].

National Offender Management Service (NOMS), Public Health England (PHE), NHS England (2013). *National Partnership Agreement Between: The National Offender Management*

Service, NHS England and Public Health England for the Co-Commissioning and Delivery of Healthcare Services in Prisons in England 2015–2016. Available from: https://assets.publishing.service.gov.uk/government/uploads/system/uploads/attachment_data/file/460445/national_partnership_agreement_commissioning-delivery-healthcare-prisons_2015.pdf [Accessed on: 2 June 2020].

Nesset, M.B., Rustad, A.B., Kjelsberg, E., Almvik, R., Bjørngaard, J.H. (2011). Health care help seeking behaviour among prisoners in Norway. *BMC Health Service Research*, 11: 301.

Offender Health Needs Assessment (2015). *Health and Justice Health Needs Assessment Toolkit for Prescribed Places of Detention*. Available from: https://assets.publishing.service.gov.uk/government/uploads/system/uploads/attachment_data/file/449652/HMP_Birmingham_HNA_West_Mids_2015.pdf [Accessed on: 2 June 2020].

Panozzo, S., Bryan, T., Collins, A., Marco, D., Lethborg, C., Philip, J.A. (2020). Complexities and constraints in end-of-life care for hospitalized prisoner patients. *Journal of Pain and Symptom Management*, DOI: 10.1016/j.jpainsymman.2020.05.24.

Peternelji-Taylor, C. (2004). An exploration of othering in Forensic Psychiatric and Correctional Nursing. *Canadian Journal of Nursing Research*, 36(4): 130–146.

Powell, J., Harris, F., Condon, L., Kemple, T. (2010). Nursing care of prisoners: staff views and experiences. *Journal of Advanced Nursing*, 66(6): 1257–1265.

Prison and Probation Ombudsman (2013). *Learning for PPO Investigations: End of Life Care*. Available from: www.ppo.gov.uk/app/uploads/2014/07/Learning_from_PPO_investigations_-_End_of_life_care_final_web.pdf [Accessed on: 2 June 2020].

Prison and Probation Ombudsman (2017). *Annual Report 2016–2017*. Available from: www.ppo.gov.uk/app/uploads/2017/07/PPO_Annual-Report-201617_Interactive.pdf [Accessed on: 2 June 2020].

Public Health England (2014). *Health and Justice Health Needs Assessment Toolkit for Prescribed Places of Detention*. Available from: https://assets.publishing.service.gov.uk/government/uploads/system/uploads/attachment_data/file/774652/Health_Needs_Assessment_Toolkit_for_Prescribed_Places_of_Detention_Part_1.pdf [Accessed on: 2 June 2020].

Public Health England (2016). *Rapid Review of Evidence of the Impact on Health Outcomes of NHS Commissioned Health Services for People in Secure and Detained Settings to Inform Future Health Interventions and Prioritisation in England*. Available from: https://assets.publishing.service.gov.uk/government/uploads/system/uploads/attachment_data/file/565231/Rapid_review_health_outcomes_secure_detained_settings.pdf [Accessed on: 2 June 2020].

Reagan, L., Shelton, D., Anderson, E. (2016). Rediscovery of self-care for incarcerated persons with diabetes. *Journal of Evidence-Based Practice in Correctional Health*, 1(1): 5.

Recio, R.S., de Agreda, J.P.A.P., Serrano, J.S. (2016). Sexually transmitted infections in male prison inmates: risk of development of new diseases. *Gaceta Sanitaria*, 30(3): 208–214.

Royal Australian College of General Practitioners (2011). *The Standards for Health Services in Australian Prisons*. 1st edition. Available from: www.racgp.org.au/FSDEDEV/media/documents/Running%20a%20practice/Practice%20standards/Health-services-in-Australian-prisons.pdf [Accessed on: 2 June 2020].

Royal College of Nursing (2009). *RCN Policy Unit Policy Briefing 14/2009. Specialist Nurses Make a Difference*. Available from: file:///C:/Users/id127162/Downloads/1409.pdf [Accessed on: 2 June 2020].

Samele, C., Forrester, A., Urquia, N., Hopkin, G. (2016). Key success and challenges in providing mental health care in an urban remand prison: a qualitative study. *Social Psychiatry and Psychiatric Epidemiology*, 51: 589–596.

Sivak, L., Cantley, L., Kelly, J., Reilly, R., Hawke, K., Mott, K., Stewart, H., McKivett, A., Rankine, S., Coulthard, A., Miller, W., Brown, A. (2017). *Model of Care for Aboriginal Prisoner Health and Wellbeing for South Australia – Executive Summary.* Adelaide, SA: Wardli-paringga Aboriginal Health Research Unit.

Solell, P., Smith, K. (2019). 'If we truly cared': understanding barriers to person-centred nursing in correctional facilities. *International Practice Development*, 9(2): 7.

Thomas, E.H., Wang, E.A., Curry, L.A., Chen, P.G. (2016). Patients' experiences managing cardiovascular disease and risk factors in prison. *Health and Justice*, 4: 4.

Turner, M., Payne, S., Barharachild, Z. (2011). Care or custody? An evaluation of palliative care in prisons in North West England. *Palliative Medicine*, 25: 370–377.

Turner, M., Peacock, M. (2017). Palliative care in UK prisons: practical and emotional challenges for staff and fellow prisoners. *Journal of Correctional Health Care*, 23(1): 56–65.

Weiskopf, C.S. (2005). Nurses' experience of caring for inmate patients. *Journal of Advanced Nursing*, 49(4): 336–343.

White, A.L., Larsson, L.S. (2012). Exploring scope of practice issues for correctional facility nurses in Montana. *Journal of Correctional Healthcare*, 18(1): 70–76.

Williams, T., Heavey, E. (2014). How to meet the challenges of correctional nursing. *Nursing*, 44(1): 51–54.

World Health Organization (WHO) (2014). *Prisons and Health.* Available from: www.euro.who.int/__data/assets/pdf_file/0005/249188/Prisons-and-Health.pdf [Accessed on: 2 June 2020].

3 Introduction to dementia

Monika Rybacka

An overview of dementia

Dementia is a syndrome caused by a number of diseases; therefore, it is an umbrella term for diseases such as Alzheimer's disease, vascular dementia or Lewy body dementia. All diseases under the umbrella of dementia involve the complex interaction of cognitive, functional, behavioural and psychological symptoms that decrease the quality of life for the person with dementia and their family members (World Alzheimer Report, 2018). It is recognised that dementia 'does not differentiate between social, economics, ethnic or geographical boundaries' (World Alzheimer Report, 2015).

The International Statistical Classification of Disease and Related Health Problems, tenth edition (World Health Organisation, 2016), provides the following clinical information and description of dementia:

> a disturbance of multiple higher cortical functions, including memory, thinking, orientation, comprehension, calculation, learning capacity, language, and judgement. Consciousness is not clouded. The impairments of cognitive function are commonly accompanied, and occasionally preceded, by deterioration in emotional control, social behaviour, or motivation.

In the UK, the National Dementia Strategy (Department of Health, 2009) describes the impact of dementia and the symptoms that may be experienced by someone diagnosed with dementia. This definition also includes the important element that dementia is a terminal illness:

> Dementia results in a progressive decline in multiple areas of function, including memory, reasoning, communication skills and the skills needed to carry out daily activities. Alongside this decline, individuals may develop behavioural and psychological symptoms such as depression, psychosis, aggression and wandering, which complicate care and can occur at any stage of the illness. . . . Dementia is a terminal condition but people can live with it for 7–12 years after diagnosis.

When reading this chapter, please remember dementia is an individual illness. Just because you've met someone with it doesn't mean that you can generalise their symptoms as dementia. The presentation of dementia for each individual is different and depends on a variety of factors including the type of dementia, their personality, life history and experiences (National Institute for Health and Care Excellence [NICE], 2006).

Incidence and prevalence of dementia

Dementia represents one of the biggest contemporary global health problems facing society (World Health Organization [WHO], 2020). The current prevalence of dementia is approximately 50 million people globally which is predicted to increase to 152 million by 2050, indicating its rapid increase across the globe. It is estimated that someone is diagnosed with dementia every three seconds, amounting to 9.9 million people every year (Alzheimer's Disease International Report, 2018). The prevalence of dementia is higher in those over the age of 65, which currently represents 7.5 per cent of the world's population and is one of the reasons for the predicted rapid increase in prevalence as the population ages (Alzheimer's Society, 2014). In the USA, those over the age of 65 are predicted to grow from 56 million in 2020 to 88 million by 2050 (Alzheimer's Association Report, 2020), and in sub-Saharan Africa, it has been estimated that those over the age of 60 will increase from 46 million people in 2015 to 157 million people by 2050 (Aboderin and Beard, 2015). In the UK, the number of people living with dementia is estimated to be over 850,000, which is predicted to rise to over one million by 2025 and two million by 2051 (WHO, 2020).

Risk factors of dementia

Unmodifiable risk factors of dementia have been identified, for example aging. Dementia is not a normal part of the aging process, but the risk of dementia doubles every five years from the age of 65 in the general population, and in those 90 years and older, the incidence of dementia continues to increase exponentially (Corrada et al., 2010). On average, there is a 1 in 6 chance of developing dementia in people over the age of 80. Aging is the most significant unmodifiable risk for developing dementia, although it is not an inevitable consequence of old age (WHO, 2020).

Another unmodifiable risk factor of dementia is ethnicity. In the US, African Americans have a higher risk of dementia, a 38 per cent increase over the span of 25 years commencing at the age of 65, followed by American Natives at 33 per cent, Latinos at 32 per cent, white Americans at 30 per cent, Asian Americans at 28 per cent and Pacific Islanders at 25 per cent (Mayeda et al., 2016). In the UK, the prevalence of dementia among Asian women was 18 per cent lower compared to white women, when the prevalence of black women was 25 per cent higher than white women, with similar representations in the prevalence of dementia in men (Pham et al., 2018).

Gender is another unmodifiable risk factor. Women are twice as likely to develop dementia as men; women are more likely to be diagnosed with Alzheimer's disease, and men with vascular dementia (Kiely, 2018). Finally genetics, a family history of dementia, genetically increases the lifetime risk of dementia to 20 per cent compared to the general public of 10 per cent (Loy et al., 2014). A small number of families have an autosomal dominant family history of early-onset dementia, and these family members have a 50 per cent chance of inheriting the mutating gene, and if they do inherit the gene, they have a lifetime dementia risk of dementia of over 95 per cent (Loy et al., 2014).

Modifiable risk factors for dementia include lifestyle choices, such as alcohol consumption, smoking, unhealthy diet and a lack of exercise. Alcohol is both a protective factor and a risk factor; light drinking has been associated with a lower risk of developing dementia, and heavy drinking has been associated with a higher risk of developing dementia compared to those who do not drink alcohol (Deng et al., 2006). A number of modifiable risk factors include a vascular component, such as smoking, eating a fatty diet and a lack of exercise. Therefore, interventions that address vascular risk factors could help reduce the risk of developing dementia and the progression of the disease once diagnosed (Peters et al., 2019). Vascular risk factors including high blood pressure, cholesterol, diabetes and obesity are more prevalent at midlife and are plausibly linked to the risk of dementia through a variety of cerebral vascular diseases, inflammatory and neurodegenerative pathways (WHO, 2020). Further protective factor for dementia are beginning to emerge such as chocolate (Cimini et al., 2013); caffeine (Eskelinen and Kivipelto, 2010); and mental stimulation, for example completing crosswords (Pillai et al., 2011).

Types of dementia

There are over 100 different types of dementia syndromes, ranging from childhood dementias, reversible dementias, non-memory related dementia and commonly known types such as Alzheimer's disease. This section will focus on the four main types of dementia: Alzheimer's disease, vascular dementia, dementia with Lewy bodies and Wernicke-Korsakoff syndrome. Among all types of dementia, Alzheimer's disease has the highest prevalence at almost 60 per cent, followed by vascular dementia at 20 per cent of people, and Lewy bodies at 15 per cent, and frontotemporal dementia at less than 5 per cent (National Institute for Health and Care Excellence [NICE], 2018).

Alzheimer's disease

Diseases under the umbrella of dementia all originate in and cause damage to the brain. Alzheimer's disease is no exception. This dementia is named after the neurologist, Dr Alois Alzheimer, who first described the disease in

1906. Dr Alzheimer reported an 'unusual disease of the cerebral cortex' to the 37th Meeting of South-West German Psychiatrists in Tubingen (Hippius and Neundorfer, 2003). He described the symptoms of a woman, which commenced when she turned 50. Auguste D.'s symptoms included memory loss, disorientation, hallucinations and ultimately her death at only 55 years. Dr Alzheimer performed a post-mortem, which showed various abnormalities of the brain. These included a thinner than normal cerebral cortex and senile plaques, previously only encountered in elderly people, along with neurofibrillary tangles (Hippius and Neundorfer, 2003). The impact of Alzheimer's disease on the brain is now often referred to as plaques and tangles, which are the build-up of amyloid plaques and neurofibrillary tangles that lead to the death of brain tissue and functioning.

Alzheimer's disease is a progressive terminal disease; as it develops, the symptoms, which are generally mild to begin with, progress to moderate and then to severe, affecting a person's ability to complete their own activities of daily living. The symptoms of Alzheimer's disease are distinct from the natural process of aging, when thinking may become slower, and some memory loss may occur. Mild, moderate and severe symptoms of Alzheimer's disease will now be described, but it must be remembered that this is an overall description of all possible symptoms and that no one person's experience of Alzheimer's disease will be the same as the next person.

Mild symptoms of Alzheimer's disease

A person with mild symptoms of Alzheimer's disease may appear to be healthy, although may have some problems of integrating with the world around them. Both the person experiencing mild symptoms and their family members often realise at this stage that there is something wrong. Common symptoms include short-term memory loss; bad decisions due to poor judgement; a lack of initiative and spontaneity; daily living tasks taking longer; asking repetitive questions; unable to pay bills or handle money; getting lost in their own neighbourhood; losing common objects; placing common objects in odd places; and mood changes, which may include increased anxiety or depression as the person struggles to cope with these symptoms. The identification of these symptoms both by the individual and their family members often leads to a diagnosis at this stage (National Institute on Aging, 2020).

Moderate symptoms of Alzheimer's disease

The symptoms increase in both severity and complexity, and the person with Alzheimer's disease will need more assistance from family members. However, family members may find this challenging. Common symptoms include increased memory loss, which leads to confusion; an inability to learn new things and to cope with new situations; difficulties with reading, writing and maths; visual difficulties, including misperception of objects; thinking may become disorganised; a shortened attention span; difficulty carrying out task with more than one step; problems with facial recognition of friends and family members; restlessness, agitation, anxiety, tearfulness and wandering, especially at dusk and in the evening; and an increase in repetitive statements or movement (National Institute of Aging, 2020).

Severe symptoms of Alzheimer's disease

When a person's Alzheimer's disease has progressed significantly, severe symptoms affect their ability to communicate and they need support with all of their activities of daily living. Alzheimer's disease is a terminal disease, but its trajectory is difficult to predict, so the end phase and the need for end-of-life care may span over weeks to months. Common severe symptoms include difficulty in swallowing, which leads to weight loss; inability to communicate; increased sleeping; inability to mobilise and may become bedridden; and loss of bowel and bladder control. The most common cause of death for people at the end stage of Alzheimer's disease is aspiration pneumonia, due to the person's inability to swallow and secretions of fluid enter the lungs, which become infected. There is currently no cure for Alzheimer's disease, although there are drugs to both treat and slow its progression (National Institute of Aging, 2020).

Vascular dementia

Vascular dementia is caused by the death of cells in the brain from a reduced blood supply due to damaged blood vessels (National Health Service, 2020). A healthy brain functions when brain cells have a constant supply of blood, which conveys oxygen and nutrients. When the blood supply is interrupted, the death of brain cells occurs. This can be caused by three main aetiological reasons. First, when narrowing of the small blood vessels occurs deep within the brain, this type of dementia is subcortical vascular dementia or small vessel disease. Second, when blood supply to a part of the brain suddenly stops due to a clot in a blood vessel, this is a stroke, and dementia that occurs after a stroke is referred to as post-stroke dementia or single-infarct dementia. Third, similar to a stroke, but incomplete strokes, transient ischaemic attacks (TIAs) can cause damage across the brain, which is referred to as multi-infarct dementia (NHS, 2020).

The early symptoms of different types of dementia vary; for example memory loss is common in the early stages of Alzheimer's disease but not common in the early stages of vascular dementia. The most common cognitive symptoms in the early stages of vascular dementia include problems with planning or organising; making decisions or solving problems; difficulties following a series of steps, such as cooking a meal; thought process may become slower; a lack of concentration; and short periods of sudden confusion. A person in the early stages of vascular dementia may also experience difficulties with recalling recent events, their speech may become less fluent and they may have difficulty with visuospatial skills (Karantzoulis and Galvin, 2011). Vascular dementia may also affect a person's mood, including apathy, depression or anxiety, possibly due to the person's insight into their difficulties. However, people with vascular dementia can become more emotionally responsive and experience extreme emotions, such as fear and anger (Ganguli, 2009).

Symptoms of vascular dementia also vary between the different types of vascular dementia. Post-stroke dementia symptoms will often be accompanied by the physical symptoms of the stroke (Novitzke, 2008). The progression of post-stroke dementia occurs in distinct stages, sometimes referred to as steps, with long periods when symptoms are stable and periods when symptoms rapidly get worse, because of additional vascular events, such as a stroke. Whereas symptoms of subcortical vascular dementia tend to gradually progress, as the area of the brain affected slowly expands (Kalaria and Erkinjuntti, 2006). Early signs of subcortical vascular dementia may include an early loss of bladder control, clumsiness, lack of facial expression and problems pronouncing words; symptoms will develop to include severe confusion or disorientation, problems with reasoning, communication and memory loss and difficulties with walking and eating (Erkinjuntti, 2007).

Dementia with Lewy bodies

Dementia with Lewy bodies (DLB) is sometimes known by other names, such as Lewy body dementia, Lewy body variant of Alzheimer's disease, diffuse Lewy body disease and cortical Lewy body disease. Lewy bodies are named after Dr Friedrich Heinrich Lewy, a German-born neurologist. In 1912, two years out of medical school and in his first year as director of the Neuropsychiatric Laboratory at the University of Breslau (now Wroclaw, Poland) Medical School, he discovered 'spherical neuronal inclusions' in the brain of a deceased Parkinson's patient (Sweeney et al., 1997). Lewy bodies are microscopic protein deposits in the brain associated with the death of brain cells. However, it is not known whether the Lewy bodies are the cause or effect of degeneration of brain cells, but they are thought to be the result of the misfolding of the protein alpha-synuclein (Gomperts et al., 2008).

Dementia with Lewy bodies (DLB) is often misdiagnosed and mistaken for Alzheimer's disease (Gaugler, 2013). However, Lewy bodies are present in people with DLB and Parkinson's disease. A significant difference between the two diseases is the location of the Lewy bodies in the brain. In Parkinson's disease, they occur in the substantia nigra which is in the mid-brain, whereas in DLB they are more widely distributed throughout the cerebral cortex. Clinically, DLB closely resembles the dementia associated with Parkinson's disease. The clinical differentiation occurs through the development of a patient's symptoms: if a patient's physical symptoms precede their cognitive symptoms by one year, this is diagnosed as Parkinson's disease; if the onset of cognitive symptoms precedes or starts at the same time as physical symptoms, DLB is diagnosed (Baba et al., 1998).

The impact DLB has on a person will depend on where the Lewy bodies are situated in the brain. If they are within the cerebellum, this will cause problems with movement similar to that of Parkinson's disease. If they are within the cerebral cortex, this will cause cognitive symptoms, although both movement and cognitive symptoms may be present simultaneously (Gomperts, 2016). DLB is a progressive condition developing over a period of several years, commencing with mild symptoms that gradually progress to affect activities of daily living. A person with DLB will usually have a combination of symptoms including those related to Alzheimer's disease and Parkinson's disease, but also symptoms unique to DLB. A unique feature of DLB is that symptoms fluctuate and a person may have a bad day or a good day, or even a bad morning and a good afternoon (Armstrong et al., 2019).

Symptoms of DLB include problems with attention and alertness; for example a person with DLB may stare into space for a long time or have periods when their speech is disorganised. Visual hallucinations occur frequently in the early stages of the condition and are often detailed and convincing, which may be very distressing. Visual misperceptions may also occur, such as mistaking a shadow or a coat on a hanger for a person (Taylor et al., 2011). Hallucinations and visual misperceptions partly explain why most people with DLB have delusions at some stage, which may include paranoia; for example there are strangers living in the house, or a spouse is having an affair or has been replaced by an identical impostor (Tsunoda et al., 2018). People may also have difficulties judging distances, and it is common to struggle with planning, organising and decision making.

Sleep disturbance is another common symptom of DLB, which includes violent movements as the person with DLB tries to act out nightmares, which is diagnosed as rapid eye movement sleep behaviour disorder (Chan et al., 2018). People with DLB will have movement difficulties when the condition is diagnosed. These symptoms are similar to those of Parkinson's disease and include slow and stiff (rigid) movement with a blank facial expression, and difficulty with their balance as their limbs may sometimes tremble (Gomperts, 2016). As the disease progresses, symptoms become similar to those of Alzheimer's disease. The life expectancy of a person with DLB varies considerably; on average, it is estimated to be from six to 12 years after the first symptoms, similar to a person with Alzheimer's disease (Gill et al., 2011).

Alcohol-related brain damage: Wernicke-Korsakoff syndrome

Alcohol-related brain damage (ARBD) is a brain disorder caused by regular consumption of large amounts of alcohol over a sustained period of time (Kopelman et al., 2009). The term ARBD covers several different conditions, including Wernicke-Korsakoff syndrome and alcoholic dementia. Neither of these conditions is considered to be a 'true' dementia, but they fall under the umbrella term of dementia as they share similar symptoms. However, the underlying causes are treatable and can halt the progression or even improve some of the symptoms of these syndromes (Kopelman et al., 2009).

People in society regularly consume higher levels of alcohol than the recommended limit. Alcohol misuse causes ARBD in a range of ways, including the impact of alcohol on nerve cells, shrinkage of brain tissue and damage to the blood vessels which causes a lack of vitamin B1 (thiamine), high blood pressure, raised cholesterol levels and an increased risk of heart attacks and strokes (Tallaksen et al., 1992). All of these conditions can damage the brain and lead to the development of other illnesses and diseases (Piano, 2017). It is important to note that not all of these factors are equally important in all forms of ARBD or in everyone with the condition. Alcohol-related brain damage leads to slightly different symptoms in different people and causes a range of conditions. The most common forms of ARBD are alcohol-related dementia and Wernicke-Korsakoff's syndrome (Ridley et al., 2013).

Korsakoff's syndrome is the most well-known form of ARBD, although is less common than other forms of ARBD such as alcoholic dementia (Ridley et al., 2013). Korsakoff's syndrome often develops as part of a condition known as Wernicke-Korsakoff syndrome. This consists of two separate but related stages: Wernicke's encephalopathy followed by Korsakoff's syndrome and Wernicke-Korsakoff syndrome, which is diagnosed in 1 in 8 people with alcoholism. However, not everyone has a clear case of Wernicke's encephalopathy before Korsakoff's syndrome develops (Oudman et al., 2014). Encephalopathy refers to permanent or temporary brain damage, disorder or disease, which affects the brain's function or structure and may be degenerative. The primary symptom is an altered mental status. Wernicke's encephalopathy usually develops suddenly, often after abrupt and untreated withdrawal from alcohol. It has a range of different symptoms, but they may not be obvious, and it can be difficult to make a diagnosis (Oudman et al., 2014).

The symptoms of Wernicke's encephalopathy can include disorientation, confusion or mild memory loss, undernutrition, involuntary jerky eye movements or paralysis of the muscles that move the eyes, poor balance or unsteadiness or other difficulties with coordinating movement (Oudman et al., 2014). If Wernicke's encephalopathy is suspected, immediate high doses of thiamine (and other B vitamins) via injection is required; prompt treatment will reverse most symptoms in a few days (Oudman et al., 2014). When Wernicke's encephalopathy is untreated, or is not treated in a timely manner, Korsakoff's syndrome develops gradually. Damage occurs in several regions of the brain including the thalamus and hypothalamus, and the cerebellum and amygdala resulting in severe loss of short-term day-to-day memory. Several other abilities may remain intact, such as working memory which is information that can be held for a short time period of time before using it (Oudman et al., 2014).

Person-centred care

Care provided to older adults and especially those with dementia, in a person-centred way, is increasingly being regarded as synonymous with the best quality care (Manthorpe and Samsi, 2016).

Person-centred care is a philosophy of care built around the needs of the individual and contingent upon knowing the person through an interpersonal relationship (Fazio et al., 2018). Kitwood (1988) applied the term person-centred care to distinguish a certain type of care approach for more medical and behavioural approaches to dementia. Kitwood focused on bringing together ideas and ways of working that emphasised communication and relationships and proposed that dementia could be best understood as an interplay between neurological impairment and psychosocial factors including health, individual psychology and the environment (Kitwood, 1988), with the rejection of a solely medical approach to dementia. Kitwood and Bredin (1992) identified that dementia does not progress in the same way for every person, and a person with dementia is in a state of relative well-being or ill-being, and there is a need for high quality personal care that affirms personhood as wonder implies recognition, respect and trust, and this is that basis for person-centred care.

Philosophically, a person with dementia needs begins with being loved at the centre surrounded by the following five key aspects: comfort, attachment, inclusion, occupation and identity (Kitwood, 1997). Individuals need comfort and warmth to 'remain in one piece' when they may feel as though they are falling apart. Individuals with dementia needs to feel attachment when they so often feel as though they are in a strange place. Individuals need to be included and involved both in care and in life, and more than simply being occupied; they need to be involved in past and current interests and sources of fulfilment and satisfaction. Finally, people with dementia need to have an identity and their families and carers must help maintain this identity (Kitwood, 1997).

Kitwood (1997) developed a conceptual approach to care that provides staff with a way of thinking about what they do according to principles that guide care and reinforce or support personhood and well-being throughout the course of dementia. Rather than simply providing care in accordance with routines organised for staff convenience, efficiency, or some other criteria, Kitwood (1997) suggested that the focus should be on the person who is the recipient of care. Kitwood's framework encourages staff to focus less on *what* is done and more on *how* it is done.

Researchers have worked to find commonalities among models and practices of person-centred dementia care. Brooker (2004) has outlined one of the most respected descriptions, which identifies four key components that are integral to a person-centred care for people with dementia and can result in a change in practice and culture. These components are: 1 valuing and respecting persons with dementia and those who care for them; 2 treating people with dementia as individuals with unique needs; 3 seeing the world from the perspective of the person with dementia, so as to understand the person's behaviour and what is being communicated, and validating the subjective experience that is being perceived as the reality of the individual; and 4 creating a positive social environment in which the person with dementia can experience relative well-being through care that promotes the building of relationships.

There has been increased recognition of how the attitudes and actions of other people, combined with their neglect, actively disempower those who have some kind of 'difference' and overlook their attempts at action and deny them a voice. This term is called social model of disability (Shakespeare and Watson, 2001). The 'social model of disability' is based on a distinction between the term's impairment and disability. In this model, the word impairment is used to refer to the actual attributes that affect a person, such as the inability to walk or breathe independently. The word disability is used to refer to the restrictions caused by society when it does not give equivalent attention and accommodation to the needs of individuals with impairments (Goering, 2015). The social model of disability identifies systemic barriers, derogatory attitudes and social exclusion, which make it difficult for individuals with impairments to engage in society (Oliver, 2013).

Kitwood (1997) theorised that some of the deteriorations in health and changes in behaviours seen in people with dementia were caused not by their diagnosis of dementia, but by how the person was being treated, receiving care or support. The term 'malignant social psychology' is used to describe a range of behaviours that undermine the personhood and well-being of people with dementia. 'Malignant social psychology' exists in relationships which involve a person living with dementia being devalued or dehumanised; for example when the person is stigmatised, or ignored, this then causes a loss of their personhood.

In the remit of a normal day spent caring for a person with dementia, it is possible to come across the use of one or probably more than one of the behaviours under 'malignant social psychology'. These types of behaviours are indicative of an abusive social culture that may be intentional or non-intentional but nevertheless exists (Smith, 2017). Its existence prohibits the provision of the positive care factors in person-centred care that are needed to provide good dementia care and invariably generates cultural ill-being. The list of types of behaviour classified as malignant social psychology are as follows:

- Treachery: using forms of deception to distract or manipulate a person or force them into compliance.
- Disempowerment: not allowing a person to use the abilities they do have, failing to help them complete actions they have initiated.
- Infantilisation: treating a person very patronisingly, as an insensitive parent might treat a young child.
- Intimidation: inducing fear in a person through the use of threats or physical power.
- Labelling: using a category such as dementia, or 'organic mental disorder' as the main basis for interacting with a person or as an excuse for their behaviour.
- Stigmatisation: treating a person as if they were a diseased object or an outcast.

- Outpacing: providing information, presenting choices at a rate too fast for the person to understand; putting the person under pressure by expecting them to do things at a rate far exceeding their current capability.
- Invalidation: failing to acknowledge the subjective reality of a person's experience and their feelings attached to it.
- Banishment: sending a person away or excluding them – physically or psychologically.
- Objectification: treating a person as if they were an object or an item of furniture rather than as the real person they are.
- Ignoring: carrying on in the presence of someone as if they were not there.
- Imposition: forcing a person to do something, overriding a desire or denying any possibility of choice.
- Withholding: refusing to give asked for attention or to meet an evident need.
- Accusation: blaming a person for actions or failures of action that arise from their inabilities or their misunderstanding of the situation.
- Disruption: intruding suddenly or disturbing upon a person's action or reflection.
- Mockery: making fun of a person's 'strange' behaviour, action or remarks, teasing or humiliating or making jokes at the person's expense.
- Disparagement: telling a person that they are incompetent, useless, worthless etc. Giving them messages, verbally or psychologically, that are damaging to their self- esteem.

The crucial point Kitwood made through the categories of malignant social psychology was how an individual would respond when experiencing, for example a care worker moving them around without explaining what was happening to them, and having a conversation with another care worker rather than the individual (objectification and ignoring) and how this could result in a decline in well-being, and even result in ill-being (Kitwood, 1997).

Changes in behaviour

Changes in behaviour can be one of the most complex aspects of caring for someone living with dementia. These behaviours usually happen when the person is feeling confused or distressed and trying to make sense of what is happening, or when they are trying to communicate that they need something. Exploring the causes of the behaviour and identifying the person's needs can help to reduce the behaviour or make the behaviour easier to manage (Ballard et al., 2011). There are several different terms used in literature and clinical settings including 'challenging behaviours', 'behaviours that challenge' and 'BPSD' (behavioural and psychological symptoms of dementia). The term 'changes in behaviour' is used to emphasise that the person living with dementia is not deliberately being 'difficult', and the behaviour can be just as challenging for the person as for those supporting them (MacKinlay and Trevitt, 2012).

It is unknown how much focal brain damage directly causes the person with dementia to behave in ways which family members and professional staff find 'challenging'. The destruction of brain cells has a role because, in most cases, the person would not have behaved in this way before the onset of their dementia. However, there may be specific reasons why the person with dementia is behaving differently, such as memory loss, language or orientation problems, changes in a person's mental and physical health, experiences of interactions with others, a sense of being out of control, frustrated with the way others are behaving or a feeling that they are not being listened to or understood (National Collaborating Centre for Mental Health, 2007). Dementia can have an impact on a person's personality and habits, which may also lead to changes in behaviour. Therefore, it is key to understand how a person with dementia will react to and deal with situations, their preferences, routines and history (Fazio et al., 2018), and by knowing and applying these 'golden nuggets', individual pieces of knowledge about a person living with dementia, appropriate care and support can be provided.

Every individual has the same basic needs, which include physical, psychological and social factors. People with dementia may be less able to recognise these needs and find it difficult to communicate what they need and therefore their behaviour may change due to trying to address and communicate these needs (Banovic et al., 2018). The following are examples of physical, psychological and social needs that may affect the behaviour, actions or mood of a person living with dementia:

Physical needs

Physical needs can include the person experiencing pain or discomfort, they may be constipated or thirsty, or in pain from an infection. The person may be on too many medications or the side effects of medication may lead to a person becoming drowsy and confused. The environment may not be supporting the person. For example, it could be too hot or too noisy, or there might not be enough for the person to do. There may be other conditions, such as sight or hearing loss, which affects a person misunderstanding or misperceiving objects in their environment. The person may be having delusions or hallucinations. These can be confusing and frightening and may affect how the person reacts to a situation (Tible et al., 2017).

Psychological needs

Psychological needs can include the person being frustrated by their situation and not being able to do the things they used to. They may be frustrated if other people assume they can't do things for themselves and take over or leave them out of decisions. The person may be depressed or anxious. They may feel threatened by an environment that doesn't seem right or familiar. They may not be able to understand and work out the world around them. Their sense of reality may be different to those around them; for example they may believe they are at their previous workplace. The person may not understand the intentions of those caring for them; for example they may see personal care as threatening or an invasion of their personal space (Cerejeira et al., 2012).

Social needs

Social needs can include the person feeling lonely or isolated. They may be bored and not have much to stimulate them or their senses (sight, hearing, touch, smell and taste). If the person has different people coming into their home, such as care workers or neighbours, they may all have their own approaches and routines, and this can be confusing. The person may be trying to 'hide' their condition from others or may not be aware of the difficulties they're having (Tible et al., 2017).

Formulation-led interventions to changes in behaviours

Approaches that are case-specific and emphasise the need for careful assessment, rather than simply trying a standard intervention are called *individualised, formulation-led approaches*. These approaches are individual intervention plans based on an understanding of the person and the surrounding factors, which could be influencing their changes in behaviour, with the inclusion of specific underlying factors that may be triggering, maintaining or exacerbating distress (Tible et al., 2017). However, evidence-based treatments and interventions need to be provided (Kim and Park, 2017). It is important to recognise that distress is not a unitary concept or a 'medical' difficulty that will resolve with standard treatment. Historically, antipsychotic drugs have been used; however, for 80 per cent of people, they were not the best 'treatment' as they did not address the underlying cause and included negative side effects (Stroup and Gray, 2018). Each person with a diagnosis of dementia will be unique in their ability to perceive, understand and communicate. Similarly, they will differ in terms of the underlying causes, triggers or maintaining factors influencing the change in behaviour they experience. In order to maximise the effectiveness of any interventions delivered, these complexities need to be understood (James, 2011).

A 'formulation' is a tool used by clinicians to relate theory to practice and can be understood as a hypothesis, or set of hypotheses to be tested (Johnstone and Dallos, 2013). Developing a formulation, requires clinicians to become inquisitive detectives, putting the pieces together to form a narrative about the person and the change in behaviour. If clinicians can develop a formulation as to why the individual is experiencing a change in behaviour, they can target interventions to tackle the underlying causes and measure whether this was effective in reducing anxiety, fear or another change in behaviour (Johnstone and Dallos, 2013).

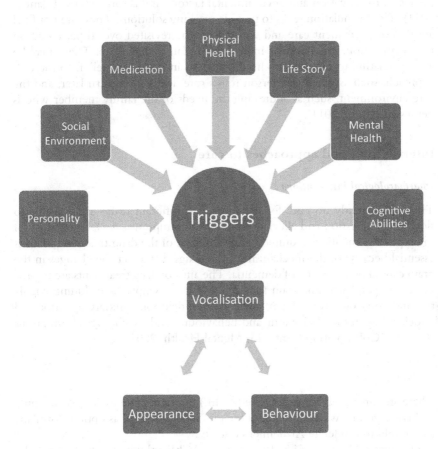

Figure 3.1 The Newcastle Clinical Model

Source: Adapted from Newcastle Model *(James, 2011)*

One such formulation-led model that can be used is the Newcastle Clinical Model (James, 2011). The model includes the range of information known to be important to consider, such as physical and mental health, the environment, as well as the life story and personality of the person, to assist in the understanding of the thoughts, emotions and beliefs underlying the person's change in behaviour.

This approach to assessment and intervention ensures that the care plan or intervention is embedded within person-centred principles and encompasses potential thoughts the person may be experiencing (Tible et al., 2017). The approach includes a functional analysis of the person's behaviour; encompasses consideration of potential unmet needs, the response/interaction of other people to the situation and environmental factors; and is carer-focused (James, 2011). The formulation seeks to provide working solutions. These are not final answers or permanent care and will need to be revisited over time. Based on this formulation, an action or intervention plan is drawn up. There may be actions relating to the person's health, such as increase pain relief, to the care approach, such as when the person resists care, leave and return later, and the care environment, such as addressing the needs of the family member who is depressed (James, 2011).

Interventions and approaches to care

Pharmacological interventions

There is currently no cure for dementia, but different drugs are available to slow the progression and alleviate some of the symptoms. A clear diagnosis of the type of dementia is required before the start of the drug treatment. This is essential because of the mechanism of the drugs that affect the changes in the brain caused by each type of dementia. The aims of drug treatments are to promote independence, maintain function and treat symptoms including cognitive and non-cognitive, such as hallucinations, delusions, anxiety, agitation and associated aggressive behaviour and behavioural and psychological symptoms (National Collaborating Centre for Mental Health, 2007).

Alzheimer's disease

There are three acetylcholinesterase (AChE) inhibitors, donepezil, galantamine and rivastigmine, which are monotherapies recommended as options for managing mild to moderate Alzheimer's disease.

Donepezil (Aricept, Eisai/Pfizer) is an AChE inhibitor, which works by increasing the concentration of acetylcholine at sites of neurotransmission. The common undesirable effects include diarrhoea, muscle cramps, fatigue, nausea, vomiting and insomnia. Galantamine (Reminyl, Shire) is an AChE inhibitor, which is similar to donepezil and also modulates activity at nicotinic receptors. The common undesirable effects include nausea and vomiting. Rivastigmine (Exelon, Novartis) is an AChE inhibitor, which is similar to donepezil and can be taken by tablet or a patch. The common undesirable effects are mainly gastrointestinal including nausea and vomiting (Casey et al., 2010).

The N-methyl-D-aspartate (NMDA) receptor antagonist memantine is a monotherapy that is recommended as an option for managing moderate to severe Alzheimer's disease. Memantine (Ebixa, Lundbeck) is a voltage-dependent, moderate-affinity, uncompetitive NMDA receptor antagonist that blocks the effects of pathologically elevated tonic levels of glutamate that may lead to neuronal dysfunction. This medication comes in both tablet and oral drop form. The common effects are dizziness, headache, constipation, somnolence and hypertension (Casey et al., 2010).

Vascular dementia

The drugs used in Alzheimer's disease are not recommended for vascular dementia, unless there is a diagnosis of mixed dementia. There are no specific drugs to treat vascular dementia; instead drug treatment for the underlying conditions is required, for example high blood pressure or high cholesterol, with the commencement or regulation of secondary prevention (Baskys and Hou, 2007). There are several non-pharmacological treatment options available.

Lewy body dementia

The three acetylcholinesterase (AChE) inhibitors donepezil, galantamine and rivastigmine, developed for treating Alzheimer's disease, are used for treating LBD's cognitive symptoms and, for some people with LBD, can reduce behavioural symptoms as well. Acetylcholinesterase (AChE) inhibitors increase brain levels of acetylcholine, a chemical important for memory and learning. In LBD, acetylcholine is in short supply; having more acetylcholine in the brain improves attention and alertness and may lessen behavioural symptoms like hallucinations. All AChE inhibitors improve cognitive and behavioural symptoms and usually do not significantly increase symptoms of parkinsonism. However, in one study of Parkinson's disease dementia, rivastigmine was associated with a mild increase in tremor in some patients (Reingold et al., 2007).

Korsakoff's syndrome

Experts recommend that anyone with a history of heavy alcohol consumption who experiences symptoms associated with Wernicke encephalopathy should be given injectable thiamine until the clinical picture is clearer (Martin et al., 2003). Once acute symptoms improve, individuals should be carefully evaluated to determine if their medical history, alcohol use and pattern of memory problems may be consistent with Korsakoff syndrome. For those who develop Korsakoff syndrome, extended treatment with oral thiamine and magnesium as well as a reduction in alcohol intake may increase chances of symptom improvement. If there is no improvement, consideration should be given to treatment of comorbid deficiencies and other medical conditions (Martin et al., 2003).

Antipsychotics

Antipsychotics are medications that are prescribed to treat hallucinations and delusions, as well as schizophrenia. Antipsychotic medications may also be helpful for anxiety and agitation and problems with mood, thinking and socialising. Most antipsychotic medications are tablets, capsules or liquid (Barnes et al., 2012). Risperidone is the only licensed medication for the short-term treatment of aggression in Alzheimer's disease, and only if aggression poses a risk or the person has not responded to non-drug approaches. Drug trials have shown that risperidone has a small but significant beneficial effect on aggression and, to a lesser extent, psychosis for people with Alzheimer's disease. These effects are seen when the drug is taken for a period of 6–12 weeks; after this time the medication can be no longer effective (Katz et al., 1999). Many people with LBD who are treated with antipsychotic medications have very severe reactions, including their symptoms becoming exacerbated, and adversely sedated and increased symptoms of parkinsonism. In rare cases, antipsychotic medications may cause a condition called 'neuroleptic malignant syndrome' which causes severe fever, muscle rigidity, kidney failure and even death (McKeith et al., 1995).

Non-pharmacological

NICE (2018) provides guidance and evidence for non-pharmacological therapies, including interventions for cognitive symptoms and maintaining function and interventions for changes in behaviour. The only non-pharmacological therapy endorsed by NICE for improving cognitive symptoms is group cognitive stimulation therapy (CST). Clare and Woods (2004) define cognitive stimulation as engagement in a range of activities and discussions (usually in a group) aimed at general enhancement of cognitive and social functioning. Typical sessions include word games, discussion of themes such as childhood and activities involving the use of the senses. A key feature of CST groups is that there are always tangible triggers to guide discussion. The aim is not to test the memory of group members but to draw out implicit memories by seeking their opinions and views. CST continually encourages new ideas, thoughts and associations, rather than just recall of previously learned information. The activities use positive aspects of reality orientation, whilst ensuring it is implemented in a sensitive and respectful manner. The activities are also designed to use generalised cognitive ability, rather than attempt to improve or rehabilitate one aspect of cognition.

Interventions endorsed by NICE (2018) associated for use in changes in behaviour include aromatherapy, massage, therapeutic use of music and/or dancing, animal-assisted therapy and multisensory stimulation.

Aromatherapy

A Cochrane review in 2014 provided an update of the evidence for aromatherapy and found that lavender was beneficial for promoting sleep. Sleep disturbance may be present in a person with dementia and improvements in the person's sleep include an increase in total sleep time and reduced requirements for sedating medication. The main positive effects of aromatherapy on people living with dementia are seen in the domains of agitation, motor activity and sleep, with no effect on cognition (Forrester et al., 2014).

Massage

Evidence suggests that there is insufficient evidence regarding the efficacy of touch or massage interventions (Hansen et al., 2006). However, there was some evidence to support the efficacy of two sub-types of touch interventions: the application of hand massage for immediate and short-term reduction of agitated behaviour and the use of touch in addition to verbal encouragement to eat (Hansen et al., 2006).

Music therapy

People with dementia may experience problems with language, however, the ability to sing is often preserved along with knowledge of song lyrics learnt in their earlier years (Bannan and Montgomery-Smith, 2008). Music therapy promotes engagement and interaction between a group using musical instruments and the voice. Music therapy encourages verbal and non-verbal expression, cognitive stimulation and listening skills and does not require any previous musical knowledge or skill.

Animal-assisted therapy

Using animals as a support tool for people with dementia has been shown to reduce stress and lower blood pressure (Raglio et al., 2013), which may be of value in patients with a vascular dementia. Evidence suggested the presence of a dog reduced aggression and agitation and increased social interaction in people with dementia (Filan and Llewellyn-Jones, 2006). Evidence also suggested that animal-assisted therapy worked better for social interaction and focusing attention in the elderly with Alzheimer's disease than in those without the condition (Danshaw-Stiles, 2001).

Multisensory stimulation

Multisensory stimulation is endorsed by NICE for people with dementia and changes in behaviour (NICE, 2006). It is thought that the multisensory stimulation approach is beneficial as it focuses on the person's sensorimotor abilities, rather than intellectual abilities which may be impaired, and may help people with dementia with changes in behaviour to be more relaxed since the stimulation often has an arousal-reducing quality. Multisensory stimulation may also help by focusing attention on external stimuli rather than on other internal needs. In addition, it may help staff interact with and see a response in people who are often thought to be unresponsive. A review of the literature found no significant effects on behaviour, mood or interactions of people with dementia. However, the review noted that the variability in how this approach is implemented and with people at different stages of dementia makes comparison across studies difficult (Sanchez et al., 2012).

Summary

Person-centredness reflects the concept of 'caring' and is underpinned by values of mutual respect, understanding for the person's and individual right to self-determination (McCormack et al., 2015). There are four main principles and features of person-centred approaches:

> Principle 1 Giving people dignity, respect and compassion.
> Principle 2 Providing coordinated care, support and treatment.
> Principle 3 Providing personalised care, support and treatment.
> Principle 4 Enabling a person.
> Lastly . . .

> A person living with dementia
> May not remember who you are
> May not remember what you said
> But they will remember how you made them feel.

References

Aboderin, I.A.G., Beard, J.R. (2015). Older people's health in sub-Saharan Africa. *Lancet*, 385: e9–e11.

Alzheimer's Association Report (2020). 2020 Alzheimer's disease facts and figures. *Alzheimer's and Dementia, The Journal of Alzheimer's Association*, 16: 391–460.

Alzheimer's Disease International Report (2018). *Dementia Statistics | Alzheimer's Disease International*. Available from: www.alz.co.uk/research/statistics [Accessed on: 22 June 2020].

Alzheimer's Society (2014). *Dementia UK Update*. Available from: www.alzheimers.org.uk/sites/default/files/migrate/downloads/dementia_uk_update.pdf [Accessed on: 22 June 2020].

Armstrong, M.J., Alliance, S., Taylor, A., Corsentino, P., Galvin, J.E. (2019). End-of-life experiences in dementia with Lewy bodies: qualitative interviews with former caregivers. *PloS One*, 14(5): e0217039.

Baba, M., Nakajo, S., Tu, P., Tomita, T., Nakaya, K., Lee, V., Trojanowski, J., Iwatsubo, T. (1998). Aggregating of x-synuclein in Lewy bodies of sporadic Parkinson's disease and dementia in Lewy bodies. *American Journal of Pathology*, 152: 4.

Ballard, C., Smith, J., Husebo, B., Aarsland, D., Corbett, A. (2011). The role of pain treatment in managing the behavioural and psychological symptoms of dementia (BPSD). *International Journal of Palliative Nursing*, 17(9): 420–424.

Bannan, N., Montgomery-Smith, C. (2008). 'Singing for the brain': reflections on the human capacity for music arising from a pilot study of group singing with Alzheimer's patients. *The Journal of the Royal Society for the Promotion of Health*, 128(2): 73–78.

Banovic, S., Zunic, L.J., Sinanovic, O. (2018). Communication difficulties as a result of dementia. *Materia Socio-Medica*, 30(3): 221–224.

Barnes, T., Banerjee, S., Collins, N., Treloar, A., McIntyre, S., Paton, C. (2012). Antipsychotics in dementia: prevalence and quality of antipsychotic drug prescribing in UK mental health services. *British Journal of Psychiatry*, 201(3): 221–226.

Baskys, A., Hou, A.C. (2007). Vascular dementia: pharmacological treatment approaches and perspectives. *Clinical Interventions in Aging*, 2(3): 327–335.

Brooker, D. (2004). What is person centred-care in dementia? *Reviews in Clinical Gerontology*, 13: 215–222.

Casey, D.A., Antimisiaris, D., O'Brien, J. (2010). Drugs for Alzheimer's disease: are they effective? *A Peer-Reviewed Journal for Formulary Management*, 35(4): 208–211.

Cerejeira, J., Lagarto, L., Mukaetova-Ladinska, E.B. (2012). Behavioral and psychological symptoms of dementia. *Frontiers in Neurology*, 3: 73.

Chan, P.C., Lee, H.H., Hong, C.T., Hu, C.J., Wu, D. (2018). REM sleep behavior disorder (RBD) in dementia with Lewy bodies (DLB). *Behavioural Neurology*, 9421098.

Cimini, A., Gentile, R., D'Angelo, B., Benedetti, E., Cristiano, L., Avantaggiati, M.L., Giordano, A., Ferri, C., Desideri, G. (2013). Cocoa powder triggers neuroprotective and preventive effects in a human Alzheimer's disease model by modulating BDNF signalling pathway. *Journal of Cellular Biochemistry*, 114(10): 2209–2220.

Clare, L., Woods, R.T. (2004). Cognitive training and cognitive rehabilitation for people with early-stage Alzheimer's disease: a review. *Neuropsychological Rehabilitation*, 14: 385–401.

Corrada, M., Brookmeyer, R., Paganini-Hill, A., Berlau, D., Kawas, C. (2010). Dementia incidence continues to increase with age in the oldest old: the 90+ study. *Annual Neurology*, 67(1): 114–121.

Danshaw-Stiles, L. (2001). Animal-assisted therapy with children and the elderly: a critical review. *Dissertation Abstracts International. Section B: The Sciences and Engineering*, 62(5–B): 4219–4224.

Deng, J., Zhou, D.H.D., Li, J., Wang, J., Gao, C., Chen, M. (2006). A 2 year follow-up study of alcohol consumption and risk of dementia. *Clinical Neurology and Neurosurgery*, 108(4): 378–383.

Department of Health (2009). *Living Well with Dementia: A National Dementia Strategy*. Available from: https://assets.publishing.service.gov.uk/government/uploads/system/uploads/attachment_data/file/168220/dh_094051.pdf [Accessed on: 22 May 2020].

Erkinjuntti, T. (2007). Vascular cognitive deterioration and stroke. *Cerebrovascular Diseases*, 24: 189–194.

Eskelinen, M.H., Kivipelto, M. (2010). Caffeine as a protective factor in dementia and Alzheimer's disease. *Journal of Alzheimer's Disease*, 20(Suppl1): S167–S174.

Fazio, S., Pace, D., Flinner, J., Kallmyer, B. (2018). The fundamentals of person-centered care for individuals with dementia. *The Gerontologist*, 58(1): 10–19.

Filan, S.L., Llewellyn-Jones, R.H. (2006). Animal-assisted therapy for dementia: a review of the literature. *International Psychogeriatrics*, 18(4): 597–611.

Forrester, L.T., Maayan, N., Orrell, M., et al. (2014). Aromatherapy for dementia. *Cochrane Database of Systematic Reviews*, 2: CD003150.

Ganguli, M. (2009). Depression, cognitive impairment and dementia: why should clinicians care about the web of causation? *Indian Journal of Psychiatry*, 51(Suppl1): S29–S34.

Gaugler, J.E., Ascher-Svanum, H., Roth, D.L., Fafowora, T., Siderowf, A., Beach, T.G. (2013). Characteristics of patients misdiagnosed with Alzheimer's disease and their medication use: an analysis of the NACC-UDS database. *BMC Geriatrics*, 13: 137.

Gill, D.P., Koepsell, T.D., Hubbard, R.A., Kukull, W.A. (2011). Risk of decline in functional activities in dementia with Lewy bodies and Alzheimer disease. *Alzheimer Disease and Associated Disorders*, 25(1): 17–23.

Goering, S. (2015). Rethinking disability: the social model of disability and chronic disease. *Current Reviews in Musculoskeletal Medicine*, 8(2): 134–138.

Gomperts, S.N. (2016). Lewy body dementias: dementia with Lewy bodies and Parkinson disease dementia. *Continuum (Minneapolis, Minn.)*, 22(2 Dementia): 435–463.

Gomperts, S.N., Rentz, D.M., Moran, E., Becker, J.A., Locascio, J.J., Klunk, W.E., Mathis, C.A., Elmaleh, D.R., Shoup, T., Fischman, A.J., Hyman, B.T., Growdon, J.H., Johnson, K.A. (2008). Imaging amyloid deposition in Lewy body diseases. *Neurology*, 71(12): 903–910.

Hansen, N.V., Jorgensen, T., Ortenbald, L. (2006). Massage and touch for dementia. *Cochrane Database Systematic Reviews*, 18(4).

Hippius, H., Neundorfer, G. (2003). The discovery of Alzheimer's disease. *Dialogues in Clinical Neuroscience*, 5(1): 101–108.

James, I.A. (2011). *Understanding Behaviour in Dementia That Challenges: A Guide to Assessment and Treatment*. London: Jessica Kingsley Publishers.

Johnstone, L., Dallos, R. (2013). *Formulation in Psychology and Psychotherapy*. London: Routledge.

Kalaria, R.N., Erkinjuntti, T. (2006). Small vessel disease and subcortical vascular dementia. *Journal of Clinical Neurology (Seoul, Korea)*, 2(1): 1–11.

Karantzoulis, S., Galvin, J.E. (2011). Distinguishing Alzheimer's disease from other major forms of dementia. *Expert Review of Neurotherapeutics*, 11(11): 1579–1591.

Katz, I.R., Jeste, D.V., Mintzer, J.E., Clyde, C., Napolitano, J., Brecher, M. (1999). Comparison of risperidone and placebo for psychosis and behavioral disturbances associated with dementia: a randomized, double-blind trial. *The Journal of Clinical Psychiatry*, 60(2): 107–115.

Kiely, A. (2018). *Why Is Dementia Different for Women?* Available from: www.alzheimers.org.uk/blog/why-dementia-different-women [Accessed on: 22 May 2020].

Kim, S.K., Park, M. (2017). Effectiveness of person-centered care on people with dementia: a systematic review and meta-analysis. *Clinical Interventions in Aging*, 12: 381–397.

Kitwood, T. (1988). The technical, the personal, and the framing of dementia. *Social Behaviour*, 3: 161–179.

Kitwood, T. (1997). *Dementia Reconsidered: The Person Comes First*. Buckingham: Open University Press.

Kitwood, T., Bredin, K. (1992). Towards a theory of dementia care: personhood and wellbeing. *Ageing Society*, 12: 269–287.

Kopelman, M.D., Thomson, A.D., Guerrini, I., Marshall, E.J. (2009). The Korsakoff syndrome: clinical aspects, psychology and treatment. *Alcohol and Alcoholism*, 44: 148–154.

Loy, C.T., Schofield, P.R., Turner, A.M., Kowk, J.B. (2014). Genetics of dementia. *Lancet*, 383: 828–840.

MacKinlay, E., Trevitt, C. (2012). *Finding Meaning in the Experience of Dementia*. London: Jessica Kingsley Publishers.

Manthorpe, J., Samsi, K. (2016). Person-centered dementia care: current perspectives. *Clinical Interventions in Aging*, 11: 1733–1740.

Martin, P., Singleton, C., Hiller – Sturmhöfel, S. (2003). The role of thiamine deficiency in alcoholic brain disease. *Alcohol Research & Health*, 27(2): 134–142.

Mayeda, E.R., Glymour, M.M., Quesenberry, C.P., Whitmer, R.A. (2016). Inequalities in dementia incidence between six racial and ethnic groups over 14 years. *Alzheimer's and Dementia Journal*, 12(3): 216–224.

McCormack, B., Borg, M., Cardiff, S., Dewing, J., Jacobs, G., Janes, N., Karlsson, B., McCance, T., Mekki, T., Porock, D., Lieshour, F., Wilson, V. (2015). Person-centredness – the 'state' of the art. *International Practice Development Journal*, 5(Suppl1).

McKeith, I., Ballard, C., Harrison, R. (1995). Neuroleptic sensitivity to risperidone in Lewy body dementia. *The Lancet*, 346: 699.

National Collaborating Centre for Mental Health (UK) (2007). *Dementia: A NICE-SCIE Guideline on Supporting People with Dementia and Their Carers in Health and Social Care. No. 42.* Available from: www.ncbi.nlm.nih.gov/books/NBK55480/ [Assessed on: 22 May 2020].

National Health Service (2020). *Vascular Dementia.* Available from: www.nhs.uk/conditions/vascular-dementia/causes/ [Accessed on: 22 June 2020].

National Institute of Aging (2020). *What Are the Signs of Alzheimer's Disease?* Available from: www.nia.nih.gov/health/what-are-signs-alzheimers-disease [Accessed on: 22 May 2020].

National Institute for Health and Care Excellence (NICE) (2006). Dementia: supporting people with dementia and their carers in health and social care. *Clinical Guideline,* 42.

National Institute for Health and Care Excellence (NICE) (2018). Dementia: assessment, management and support for people living with dementia care. *Clinical Guideline,* 97. Available from: https://www.nice.org.uk/guidance/ng97/resources/dementia-assessment-management-and-support-for-people-living-with-dementia-and-their-carers-pdf-1837760199109 [Accessed on: 17 October 2020].

Novitzke, J. (2008). Privation of memory: what can be done to help stroke patients remember? *Journal of Vascular and Interventional Neurology,* 1(4): 122–123.

Oliver, M. (2013). The social model of disability: thirty years on. *Disability & Society,* 28(7): 1024–1026.

Oudman, E., Van der Stigchel, S., Postma, A., Wijnia, J.W., Nijboer, T.C. (2014). A case of chronic Wernicke's encephalopathy: a neuropsychological study. *Frontiers in Psychiatry,* 5: 59.

Peters, R., Booth, A., Rockwood, K., et al. (2019). Combining modifiable risk factors and risk of dementia: a systematic review and meta-analysis. *BMJ Open,* 9: e022846.

Pham, T.M., Petersen, I., Walters, K., Raine, R., Manthorpe, J., Mukadam, N., Cooper, C. (2018). Trends in dementia diagnosis rates in UK ethnic groups: analysis of UK primary care data. *Clinical Epidemiology,* 10: 949–960.

Piano, M.R. (2017). Alcohol's effects on the cardiovascular system. *Alcohol Research: Current Reviews,* 38(2): 219–241.

Pillai, J.A., Hall, C.B., Dickson, D.W., Buschke, H., Lipton, R.B., Verghese, J. (2011). Association of crossword puzzle participation with memory decline in persons who develop dementia. *Journal of the International Neuropsychological Society,* 17(6).

Raglio, A., Bellandi, D., Baiardi, P., et al. (2013). Listening to music and active music therapy in behavioural disturbances in dementia: a crossover study. *Journal of the American Geriatrics Society,* 61(4): 645–647.

Reingold, J.L., Morgan, J.C., Sethi, K.D. (2007). Rivastigmine for the treatment of dementia associated with Parkinson's disease. *Neuropsychiatric Disease and Treatment,* 3(6): 775–783.

Ridley, N.J., Draper, B., Withall, A. (2013). Alcohol-related dementia: an update of the evidence. *Alzheimer's Research & Therapy,* 5(1): 3.

Sanchez, A., Millan-Calanti, J., Lorenzo-Lopez, L., Maseda, A. (2012). Multisensory stimulation for people with dementia: a review of the literature. *American Journal of Alzheimer's Disease & Other Dementiasr,* 28(1): 7–14.

Shakespeare, T., Watson, N. (2001). The social model of disability: an outdated ideology in exploring theories and expanding methodologies: where are we and where do we need to go? *Research in Social Science and Disability,* 2: 9–28.

Smith, P. (2017). *Dementia Care – The Adaptive Response: A Stress Reductionist Approach.* Oxford: Routledge.

Stroup, T.S., Gray, N. (2018). Management of common adverse effects of antipsychotic medications. *World Psychiatry: Official Journal of the World Psychiatric Association,* 17(3): 341–356.

Sweeney, P., Lloyd, M., Daroff, R. (1997). What's in a name? Dr. Lewey and the Lewy body. *Neurology*, 49(2): 629–630.

Tallaksen, C., Bohmer, T., Bell, H. (1992). Blood and serum thiamine and thiamine phosphate esters concentrations in patients with alcohol dependence syndrome before and after thiamine treatment. *Alcoholism: Clinical and Experimental Research*, 16: 320–325.

Taylor, J.P., Firbank, M., Barnett, N., Pearce, S., Livingstone, A., Mosimann, U., Eyre, J., McKeith, I.G., O'Brien, J.T. (2011). Visual hallucinations in dementia with Lewy bodies: transcranial magnetic stimulation study. *The British Journal of Psychiatry*, 199(6): 492–500.

Tible, O.P., Riese, F., Savaskan, E., von Gunten, A. (2017). Best practice in the management of behavioural and psychological symptoms of dementia. *Therapeutic Advances in Neurological Disorders*, 10(8): 297–309.

Tsunoda, N., Hashimoto, M., Ishikawa, T. (2018). Clinical features of auditory hallucinations in patients with dementia with Lewy bodies: a soundtrack of visual hallucinations. *Journal of Clinical Psychiatry*, 79(3): 17m11623.

World Alzheimer Report (2015). *The Global Impact of Dementia: An Analysis of Prevalence, Incidence, Cost and Trends*. London: Alzheimer's Disease International.

World Alzheimer Report (2018). *The State of the Art of Dementia Research: New frontiers*. London: Alzheimer's Disease International.

World Health Organization (WHO) (2016). *ICD-10: International Statistical Classification of Diseases and Related Health Problems: Tenth Revision*. Available from: www.who.int/classifications/icd/icdonlineversions/en/ [Accessed on: 24 May 2020].

World Health Organization (WHO) (2020). *Dementia*. Available from: www.who.int/newsroom/fact-sheets/detail/dementia [Accessed on: 22 June 2020].

4 Dementia in prison

Joanne Brooke

Dementia in prison

The opening section of this chapter will explore the prevalence and incidence of dementia in prison populations. It will then discuss some of the issues with current estimates, the barriers and challenges of diagnosing a prisoner with dementia in the prison setting and the importance of screening prisoners at an earlier age because of their increased risk factors of developing a dementia.

Prevalence and incidence of dementia in prison

The prevalence of dementia in prison has been estimated through a number of individual studies within different countries and two systematic reviews that provide an overview of this data. Both approaches will be discussed. The prevalence of dementia in prison from individual studies has been estimated to range from 0.8 per cent to 18.8 per cent (Brooke et al., 2020). In France, evidence suggests that about one-fifth of older prisoners have a dementia (Combalbert et al., 2018). Similar results have been identified across four prisons within England, with 12 per cent of older prisoners demonstrating cognitive impairment and 0.8 per cent severe dementia (Kingston et al., 2011). A review of nine individual studies exploring the prevalence of dementia in prison found 3.3 per cent of older prisoners had dementia, and 11.8 per cent had cognitive impairment (di Lorito et al., 2018). Four of these studies were completed in the USA (Koenig et al., 1995; Regan et al., 2002; Caverley, 2006; Williams et al., 2012), four in the UK (Fazel et al., 2001; Murdoch et al., 2008; Kingston et al., 2011; Hayes et al., 2012) and one in France (Combalbert et al., 2016).

In the UK, estimates do vary as they have also identified 5 per cent of prisoners aged over 55 are likely to have a dementia, but not necessarily diagnosed with dementia (Moll, 2013). This discrepancy may be explained by the design of studies, as studies screening prison populations found a disparity of those with a diagnosis of dementia (2 per cent) compared to those with a suggested cognitive impairment (12.8–18.8 per cent) (Shepherd et al., 2017; Combalbert et al., 2018). A further difference between the results of estimated prevalence of dementia across these studies may be due to the population explored and screened and the diagnostic tools applied to screen for dementia. The population explored by Shepherd et al. (2017) in Australia was specifically the Aboriginal and Torres Strait Islander prisoners, and therefore applied a culturally appropriate cognitive screening tool, the Kimberley Indigenous Cognitive Assessment Tool [KICA] (LoGiudice et al., 2006). Whereas, Combalbert et al. (2018) applied the Mini Mental State Examination [MMSE] (Folstein et al., 1975). The importance of which cognitive screening tool may not be of a concern, as all of these cognitive screening tools may not be appropriate for a prison population. For example the first elements on the MMSE assess orientation include the year, month, day, date and time. However, due to the impact of the prison environment and regime, many prisoners without cognitive impairment become disorientated (Grassian, 2008).

Barriers and challenges of diagnosing dementia in a prison setting

The use of appropriate screening tools in diagnosing dementia in a prison setting poses barriers and challenges. A cognitive screening tool has been developed in the USA to specifically assess the prison activities of daily living (PADLs), which evaluates the following commands: dropping to the floor for alarms, standing for head counts, ambulating to the dinner hall for meals, hearing orders from staff and climbing up and down from the top bunk (Williams et al., 2009). However, it is unsure how this would translate to other prison regimes around the world, especially in England and Wales. Healthcare professionals have also identified the need for specific cognitive screening tools appropriate for the prison setting, as current tools have been found lacking and unlikely to identify new cases of dementia (Williams et al., 2012; Patterson et al., 2016). Recommendations from healthcare professionals working in the prison environment include a simple memory test and a cognition test, and if a prisoner fails one or both of these tests, then further cognitive screening by psychiatrists would be appropriate (Patterson et al., 2016). The issue of identifying the early stages of dementia in prison supports current studies that suggest a diagnosis of dementia during a prison sentence occurs in the later stages of the disease (Gaston, 2018).

Prisoners' increased risk factors

Prisoners are at an increased risk of developing dementia. One reason is the fact that prisoners are acknowledged to have an accelerated aging process, which has been described as their physiological health being ten years, or more recently 15 years advanced of their chronological age (Grant, 1999; Kouyoumdjian et al., 2017). Prisoners' accelerated aging has been contributed to poor health and life choices prior to their prison sentence, which continue during their sentence because of a lack of support and understanding of the impact of their choices on their health (Maschi et al., 2012; Williams et al., 2012). Therefore, prisoners have been identified to develop long-term health conditions at an earlier age that those living in the community (Sharupski et al., 2018). The prevalence of long-term health conditions in prisoners aged 50–54 in the UK has been estimated to be over 71 per cent and in those aged over 70, this increases to 92 per cent (Hayes et al., 2012). Long-term health conditions such as hypertension, diabetes, high cholesterol and heart disease are all associated with an increase in the risk of developing a dementia (Corrada et al., 2017; Ojo and Brooke, 2015; Wolters et al., 2018). This is alongside the risk of dementia, as identified in the general population, which doubles every five years from the age of 65 (Corrada et al., 2010).

Further risk factors for developing a dementia within the prison population may include lower educational attainment, low socio-economic status, increased rates of psychiatric morbidities and traumatic brain injuries; and with living in a prison, the risk factor of poor nutrition and a lack of exercise are important to consider (Maschi et al., 2012; Williams et al., 2012). Risk factors of dementia identified in the general population also need to be considered and include earlier life depression, smoking, lack of physical and intellectual activities and socialisation, especially socialisation in later life (Byers and Yaffe, 2011; Reitz et al., 2007; Ruthirakuhan et al., 2012; Fratiglioni et al., 2004). All of these require the implementation of initiatives, services, screening and health checks for older prisoners.

Living in prison with dementia

This section is divided into two main elements and will commence with a discussion regarding the implementation of person-centred dementia care and support within prison settings, and the current barriers and challenges of this approach. The following section will explore past failures in supporting prisoners with dementia through the examination of fatal incidents, and the learning and changes to practice that have since occurred.

Person-centred dementia care and support in prison

The implementation of person-centred dementia care as defined by Kitwood (1997) and discussed in Chapter 3 should be implemented in all institutional settings which support people with dementia and this includes prison settings. Four elements related to the successful implementation of person-centred dementia care in prison will be discussed in further detail. These four elements are comparable with those identified to support the social needs of older prisoners, and therefore there is a clear need to address them with the implementation of appropriate initiatives. The four elements include the environment, education for prison staff, meaningful engagement and a collaborative approach to support (Lee et al., 2016; du Toit and McGrath, 2018).

The environment

There are significant differences in the physical environment of prisons around the world. In England and Wales, the differences in prisons range from HMP Wakefield, which was originally built in 1594, although most of the buildings now date from the Victoria Era, and HM Prison Berwyn, which was purposed built with a focus on rehabilitation of prisoners and opened in 2017. In England and Wales, older prisons built in or before the Victorian Era currently hold the majority of prisoners. However, there is an emphasis on building new and appropriate environments to support the rehabilitation of prisoners. The environment has a negative impact on older prisoners and those with dementia, including the inability to climb stairs, navigate poorly lighted areas, and uneven floors (Bedard et al., 2016; Human Rights Watch, 2012). Similar difficulties have been identified in Australia, such as climbing onto a top bunk and passing through narrow doorways with walking aids or wheelchairs (Baidawi et al., 2011). Adaptations to old prisons are occurring; for example within their Enhanced Care Unit, the Jefferson City Correctional Centre, in Missouri, USA, has adapted the environment to accommodate wheelchairs, alongside the installations of handrails in toilets and showers (Brown, 2015).

A comprehensive programme for prisoners with dementia, which included environmental adaptations, is the Special Needs Program for Inmate-Patients with Dementia (SNPID, Hodel and Sanchez, 2012). The SNPID is described in more depth in a later section. The environmental adaptations included coloured name plates on cell doors; the walls within cells were painted a different colour around the toilet to differentiate the toileting and sleeping areas; pictures over the sink of someone washing their hands; and the implementation of a number of large calendars, showing the dates, routine events and pictorial information of the weather and appropriate clothes to wear. Outside the cell, adaptations included smaller tables and more time allowed for dining. In the UK, the concept of dementia-friendly prisons has been explored (Treacy et al., 2019), the Dementia Friendly Physical Environment Checklist (Dementia Action Alliance, 2018) was applied to specialist units for older prisoners and those with dementia that had been adapted with stair lifts and quiet rooms. These wings were found to be easier to navigate and more comfortable. However, they did not meet the standards of 'dementia friendliness', for example cell doors were too narrow to accommodate wheelchairs. Therefore, the physical environments of many prisons still need to be addressed to adequately support both older prisoners and those with dementia.

Education for prison staff

The complex health and social needs of older prisoners and those with dementia require consistent care and support, which create unique challenges for prison staff, and health and social care provision (Wangmo et al., 2015). An important element for prisoners with dementia is the ability of staff to recognise and support, rather than reprimand behaviours that may challenge the regime within the prison (Carpenter and Dave, 2004). Previously, prison officers have suspected a dementia in five times as many prisoners as healthcare professionals (Williams et al., 2009). Currently both prison staff and health and social care professionals have reported difficulties in identifying the difference between dementia, mental health conditions and psychotic episodes because of illegal drug use in the prison setting (Gaston, 2018; Dillon et al., 2018). Dementia education has occurred in the prison setting but only for specific staff within dementia initiatives (Hodel and Sanchez, 2012), or as a topic within a wider workshop on supporting older prisoners (Masters et al., 2016).

Dementia education within prison settings, which incorporates prison staff, prisoners, health and social care professionals and all external agencies, is essential. The development of prison officer's knowledge has commenced in the UK (McCrudden and Sindano, 2016; Gray, 2018). A recent study has addressed the wider issue of dementia education across all staff and external agencies (Brooke and Rybacka, 2020). A prison-specific dementia education workshop was developed from prison staff, prisoners and external agencies' knowledge and experiences of supporting prisoners with dementia. The workshop aimed to develop knowledge of dementia in the prison setting among prison staff, prisoners, and health and social care professionals to enable and empower staff and prisoners to support a prisoner with dementia. However, Brooke and Rybacka (2020) identified that training alone would not be sufficient to change practices, environments and regimes to effectively support prisoners with dementia.

Meaningful/purposive engagement

Initiatives within prison settings have focused on the rehabilitation and training of younger prisoners to support them on release and enable them to find employment. However, these are not suitable or appropriate for older prisoners. A consideration of older prisoners' needs and how to improve the quality of care for prisoners with dementia is required and has been explored by prison healthcare professionals (Williams et al., 2012; Patterson et al., 2016) and identified through interviews and case note reviews, as well as the application of validated cognitive and forensic need assessments (Hayes et al., 2012; Shepherd et al., 2017). The evidence from these studies has led to the development and implementation of meaningful and purposive initiatives for prisoners over the age of 55, which are discussed in the last section of this chapter.

A collaborative approach to support

There is a need for a collaborative approach of shared responsibility and provision of support to ensure the safety of older prisoners and those with dementia; this includes prison staff, health and social care professionals, external agencies and fellow prisoners (Brown, 2015). A collaborative approach is needed within a cohesive framework to enable the identification, assessment and support of older prisoners and those with dementia (Williams et al., 2012; Patterson et al., 2016). Essential elements of a cohesive framework would include the development of an appropriate cognitive screening tool, a multidisciplinary approach, services and initiatives specifically for older prisoners and those with dementia. However, this also needs to occur alongside an equitable approach to support older prisoners and those with dementia to access generic services for all prisoners (Brooke et al., 2020).

Examination of dementia in prison through fatal incidents

The Prison and Probation Ombudsman (2016) explored three elements of the support required by prisoners with dementia through the examination of case studies of fatal incidents, which highlighted the need for improvement in the three areas of dementia and decision making, responsibilities and neglect, and caring for those with dementia.

Dementia and decision making

The first case study described the events of a 79-year-old man admitted to prison for the first time with an existing diagnosis of diabetes, heart failure and dementia. Four years into his sentence, he had significantly declined and was transferred to a specialist unit for older prisoners with long-term medical conditions. On admission to the unit, a full assessment was completed, which highlighted the prisoner did not have the mental capacity to inform decisions regarding care and treatment. Therefore, according to the Mental Capacity Act (2005), a referral for an advocate to support decision making was completed, but prior to the appointment of an advocate, the prisoner collapsed. The staff were unsure whether they should begin resuscitation, which they did. However, this was unsuccessful, and the prisoner died.

This case study highlights the gradual decline of dementia, which affects a person's mental capacity to make informed decisions. In England and Wales, the Mental Capacity Act (2005) is a legal framework implemented by the government, which defines the laws of acting and deciding for an adult who lacks the mental capacity to make decisions. It has five statutory principles, the first being the presumption that the person has capacity until proven otherwise. The Mental Capacity Act (2005) defines a person as lacking mental capacity if they are unable to process the information given to them to make an informed decision. This includes understanding the information; being able to retain the information; being able to debate the pros and cons of the information; and finally being able to communicate their decision either verbally, in writing, through sign language, blinking or squeezing of a hand.

The second statutory principle of the Mental Capacity Act (2005) is to ensure individuals are supported to make their own decisions; even if they lack the capacity, they should still be involved in the decision-making process, which includes people and prisoners with dementia. The third principle, which is not applicable in this case, states that people who have the mental capacity have the right to make unwise conditions. Again, this will include people with dementia if they have the mental capacity to make these decisions. The last two statutory principles inform the decisions for a person who lacks mental capacity: they must be in the person's best interest and be the least restrictive option to support the person's rights and freedom.

The situation described in this case study could have been avoided if advance directives had been in place. Advance directives are sometimes referred to as advance care planning or a living will, which may include the decision to refuse treatment (Harding, 2015). Advance directives for a person with dementia are imperative to ensure the person's values and preferences regarding medical care, treatment and end-of-life decisions are respected (Porteri, 2018). The implementation of advance directives for a person with dementia is complex, as treatment options and end-of-life care need to be considered early in the progression of the disease, when the person has the mental capacity to engage in these difficult and complex conversations. Frameworks have been developed to support these conversations, such as a goal-directed Dementia-Specific Advance Directive (Gaster et al., 2017).

The recommendation in this case study to include the implementation of advance directives is further complicated by a lack of routine practice in the community of discussing end-of-life decisions with people in the early stages of dementia and their family members; so, it is unlikely that people entering prison with a diagnosis of dementia will have an advance directive in place. Barriers for the creation and implementation of advance directives in the community have been identified, including a lack of understanding of advance directives by people with dementia, their families and healthcare professionals (Schmidhuber et al., 2017; Poppe et al., 2013; Brooke and Kirk, 2014; Dening et al., 2011). Alongside these is the difficulty in finding the 'right time' to begin these conversations and the reluctance and avoidance of both people with dementia and their family members to commence these sensitive and distressing conversations, at a time when the person with dementia is living well (van der Steen et al., 2014; de Vleminck et al., 2014; Dickinson et al., 2013; Robinson et al., 2013). These conversations and decision-making processes will become more difficult as a person enters prison, away from any friends or family and in a stressful environment that will affect the progression of their dementia.

Responsibilities and neglect

This case study described the events of a 63-year-old man admitted to prison, with a medical history of a series of strokes, which led to the diagnosis of vascular dementia. On admission to prison, a full physical assessment was completed and he was placed on a disability care plan. During his prison sentence, his condition deteriorated and he did not always take his medication or address his hygiene needs. The prisoner complained of painful feet, and although a doctor suggested the need for a podiatrist to visit him, the healthcare manager informed the investigation that the prisoner would need to complete a written application to request a visit from a podiatrist. However, the prisoner did not have the mental capacity to complete this process, and the Prison and Ombudsman (2016) found this to be a case of neglect. However, this is an investigation of fatal incidents; when the prisoner required end-of-life care, he was transferred to a hospital with an escort and restrained. Once at the hospital, the prisoner remained restrained for three days and died two days following the removal of the restraints. The Prison and Ombudsman (2016) found there had been a lack of an appropriate risk assessment that took into account his current health situation and the lack of mobility of this prisoner from his previous strokes.

Since this case study, in England and Wales the Prison Service Instruction (PSI) Adult Social Care 03/2016 has been implemented. This PSI 03/2016 supports the Care Act (2014) in England, and the Social Services and Well-being Act (2014) in Wales. Both acts define local social care authorities have the responsibility to complete assessments of individual prisoners, with the aim of preventing an escalation of needs; providing information, advice and aids to support activities of daily living to support independence; and the provision of social care when required. The PSI 03/2016 also addresses communication, identification and referral process, with an emphasis on prisoner self-report, but also the responsibilities of the prison to communicate with local authorities when prison staff identify a prisoner may have care and support needs. Importantly, the PSI 03/2016 identifies the prison's responsibility to inform the local authority regarding the need to appoint an advocate for a prisoner who may lack the mental capacity to support informed decisions regarding assessment, treatment and care plans.

The Care Act (2014) emphasises the importance of the implementation of a professional lead for older prisoners, and in 2014 this had been implemented in 81 per cent of prisons in England and Wales. However, statutory social care for prisoners was still not being provided because of a lack of understanding of statutory social care and who would be responsible for the provision of this care (O'Hara et al., 2015). Following the Care Act (2014), a number of models for the provision of social care for the prison setting have been identified, of which a combination has been found essential (Lee et al., 2016). The first model identified was the accommodation and adaptation of the prison setting, which again returns to the necessity to adapt old prisons to support prisoners with mobility difficulties. However, this requires significant redevelopment and substantial cost. The second model is that of regime adaptation, with the provision of initiatives specifically for older prisoners outside of the usual prison regime, such as the comprehensive programme of True Grit (Harrison, 2006; Kopera-Frye et al., 2013), which will be discussed in more depth in the next section. This model has been widely implemented but to date not robustly evaluated.

The third model was the implementation of informal and formal carers. The use of peer support within the prison setting has increased in recent years because of the increase of older prisoners with complex needs. A comprehensive peer support programme implemented to support prisoners with dementia is Gold Coats (Berry et al., 2016). Similar initiatives exist in the UK; for example prisoners with dementia receive formal training and support from the Buddy Support Worker (Resettlement and Care of Older ex-Offenders [RECOOP], 2019). Both initiatives are explored in further detail in the following section. Peer support has been associated with positive health outcomes for those providing care and support, and a method to alter their life narratives, alongside a positive effect on the prisoners receiving the care (Stewart, 2018). However, there is no evidence to support the cost-effectiveness of the provision of social care through the model of peer support (South et al., 2014). The fourth model was extending the role of healthcare professionals. This model suggests the development of healthcare provision, which already exists to support prisoners social care needs. This has been suggested as the most straightforward model, but not necessarily the best, model to adopt (Lee et al., 2016).

The final element in this case study was that of restraint of an elderly prisoner, with a medical history of several strokes, vascular dementia and requiring end-of-life care. The rules and procedures regarding escorting unwell prisoners to hospitals in England and Wales have been revised in 2015 and include those who are terminally ill. The focus on the transfer of terminally ill prisoners to hospital is essential, due to the increase of deaths in prison custody in England and Wales, which has increased from 1.1 per 1,000 prisoners in 2007 to 2.2 per 1,000 in 2017, of which 62.7 per cent were from natural causes (Ministry of Justice, 2017). The Prison and Probation Ombudsman first addressed this issue in 2013 and stated: 'While a prison's first duty is to protect the public, too often restraints are used in a disproportionate, inappropriate, and sometimes inhuman ways'. (p. 5). Since this statement, the Prison Service Instruction 33/2015 has addressed the restraints of terminally ill prisoners during transfer to the hospital, which discusses the balance of security against clinical needs of the prisoner, and the need to clarify the distinction between the risk of harm by or escape of the prisoner when well and the risk posed due to their current health condition. However, this case study demonstrated these instructions are not robust enough to prevent restraints of a terminally ill prisoner on transfer to the hospital, or whilst a patient is in the hospital.

Caring for those with dementia

This case study described the events of a 63-year-old man who began his sentence with a medical history of heart disease, hypertension and diabetes. During his sentence, he had a number of falls and was advised not to leave his cell. The prison staff began to raise concerns about his memory, as his speech appeared slower and he was no longer able to follow a conversation. He was diagnosed with dementia. The prisoner was appropriately assessed by both health and social care professionals but refused all support from them; instead he accepted the support of fellow prisoners. Eventually, one prisoner became his carer and supported him with activities such as getting dressed, collecting his meals and washing his clothes. The support was provided with normality and dignity until the prisoner died at the age of 73 (Prison and Ombudsman, 2016).

The peer support provided in this case study is successful and met the need of the prisoner. Examples of peer support and the training prisoners receive to provide care and support are discussed in relation to dementia in more depth in the following section. Peer support is a model of care for older prisoners with complex health conditions, including dementia (Lee et al., 2016), and is a recurrent theme throughout this chapter. Peer support programmes not only care and support older prisoners and those with dementia but address the vulnerabilities of these prisoners, such as increased isolation and a lack of socialisation (Brown, 2015) due to bullying and harassment from other prisoners (Wilson and Barboza, 2010). However, although the Care Act (2014) has potentially addressed this issue, it also needs to be acknowledged that even if a prisoner is accepting of social care, gaining the necessary social care for older prisoners and those with dementia in prison is difficult (O'Hara et al., 2015).

Initiatives to support prisoners with dementia

The emphasis of this section is initiatives to support older prisoners and those with dementia. The focus is on older prisoners, as most initiatives are specifically commenced for older prisoners, and then encompass prisoners with dementia. These will be discussed under a number of subheadings which describe the type of support provided, including peer support, specific units and purposive initiatives. This will be followed by a discussion of the wider issue of evaluation and dissemination of these programmes, which has occurred through the media and grey literature, without robust evaluations or measurement of expected or appropriate outcomes.

1 Peer support

Peer support volunteer programmes are increasing in prisons because of the needs of older prisoners, including those with dementia and those reaching the end of their life. Prisoners as caregivers, as highlighted earlier in this chapter, provide the opportunities for prisoners to engage in these programmes, which supports them to alter their life narrative (Stewart, 2018), through a process of developing positive self-identify (Cloyes et al., 2014). Prisoner peer support not only benefits the prisoners providing support but also those receiving support and the prison community (Stewart and Edmond, 2017). Two peer support programmes, which support prisoners with dementia, include the Gold Coats in the USA (Belluck, 2012; Berry et al., 2016) and the Buddy Support Worker in England (RECOOP, 2019).

The Gold Coats

In California Men's Colony, a minimum- to medium-security male prison, the Gold Coats programme was created and implemented to train and support prisoners to learn the necessary skills to support older prisoners with cognitive impairment and dementia (Berry et al., 2016). The term 'Gold Coat' refers to the colour of the smock worn by prisoners who have completed the programme and successfully passed the Gold Coat training. The role of a Gold Coat is not only to support and care for another prisoners, but also to protect them from bullying and victimisation by other prisoners (Belluck, 2012). There is an extensive interview process for those prisoners who are interested in becoming a Gold Coat, who must also meet the inclusion criteria of no disciplinary action within prison for the past ten years; a long sentence remaining or a life sentence; following assessment, no history of a current cognitive or emotional problems; and a history of rehabilitative and community service within the current sentence in prison.

The Gold Coats training programme is delivered by a member of the psychology team within the prison, usually the staff psychologist. The training ranges from 90 to 120 days, which involves a review and follow-up. The training programme explores how to care for and support a cognitively impaired client (fellow prisoner) through sessions on functional presentation; effective communication; responding to irritability and anger; how to redirect or de-escalate situations; cognitive focusing techniques; cognitive exercises; assisting with activities of daily living; coaching physical exercise and sports activities; providing social support and recreational activities; providing companionship at meals, and other activities and events; and accessing prison resources and assisting in letter writing. This comprehensive list, with a focus on supporting prisoners with dementia allows Gold Coats to address these prisoners' health and social needs and to slow the progression of their cognitive impairment. However, there are limits on Gold Coats' responsibilities, and they cannot complete activities that constitute a professional caregiving responsibility.

A quote from a Gold Coat demonstrates how this programme supported both the Gold Coats and their clients, and the emotional impact of taking on this role:

> My first client was an angry, disabled patient who would not eat. Staff tried to bribe him to eat but it only made him angry. I sat with him and he finally said he liked coffee. I was able to get hem coffee but told him he had to eat a little first. He did and then started eating regularly. We became very close and I cared for him for a long time – I cleaned up when he soiled himself, helped him shower etc. all the while trying to protect his dignity. Eventually, he ended up in the hospice, where I continued to visit him. Just before he passed, he told me 'thank you for everything.' I cried like a baby.
>
> (Berry et al., 2016, p. 65)

Buddy Support Worker

In the UK, the Buddy Support Worker has been introduced in the geographical location of prisons clustered in the South West of England. Younger prisoners, who are eligible can apply to begin the training programme to become a Buddy Support Worker. This initiative is led by RECOOP, whilst working closely with each prison and their health and social care providers. The training programme has been adapted from the National Care Certificate, which encompasses the standards for health and social care workers in England. The standards are the basis for each module of the training programme and include understanding your role and personal development; duty of care; equality and diversity; working in a person-centred way; communication and advocacy skills; privacy and dignity, fluids and nutrition; safeguarding adults; health and safety; handling information; cleaning and infection prevention/control; assisting someone in a wheelchair; awareness of mental health, dementia and learning disabilities; and health and healthy aging (RECOOP, 2019). Unlike the Gold Coats, a Buddy Support Worker provides social support and not personal hygiene; there is a strict rule of nothing between a client's nipples to knees.

Prisoners need to complete and pass each module and are chaperoned providing support to older prisoners before becoming a Buddy Support Worker. One buddy explained the in-depth approach to becoming a buddy:

> There is a probation period where they (trainers) do come out and check you are doing it right, I had to get a written statement from one of my clients (fellow prisoner), and from one of the officers, so you are supervised for the first couple of months.
>
> (Brooke and Jackson, 2019, p. 813)

However, the training of each Buddy Support Worker continues, with monthly meetings, where they are able to discuss their concerns, difficulties and best practice. This was an important element to support buddies to discuss the care and support of each client, with both other buddies and prison staff, which was viewed as essential as the buddies were a changing group of prisoners, as either being transferred to another prison or completing their sentence. As one buddy stated:

> It is about best practice; we tell each other what we have been doing, what is working well for us because at the end of the day if I get shipped out to a different jail they have got to step in, it kind of alleviates the teething problems.
>
> (Brooke and Jackson, 2019, p. 814)

The buddy support worker training programme supported buddies to understand dementia and the provision of person-centred care. One buddy provided insight into person-centred care for a client with dementia, and discussed when to step in and help and when to stand back to support the prisoner's independence with respect and dignity.

> I will stand at the door and watch, yesterday he was trying to make his bed he got the sheet and the pillow done, but he put the orange blanket the wrong way round, and he was moving it up the bed and it was coming up and he was moving it down and it was going down, so I went in and said 'do you want a hand with that' and he let me finish it off, but maybe next time he might just get it right. It is so they don't lose their dignity.
>
> (Brooke and Jackson, 2019, p. 814)

The success of the Buddy Support Worker has been acknowledged through an award from the Health Service Journal Patient Safety Awards in 2019, when the scheme was independently judged by experts from across the health and social care sector.

2 Specific units

Prisons around the world are developing their provision for older prisoners with complex health needs, including dementia. One element has been the development of High Dependency Units (Brown, 2015; Brooke, 2018) and the Special Needs Program for Inmate-Patients with Dementia (Hodel and Sanchez, 2012). The cost benefit of these initiatives within a system that had financial restraints is still to be realised. Specialist older prisoner units are projected to be more expensive, by 17 per cent, than housing older prisoners with complex health needs within the general prison population (Maschi et al., 2012). However, the success of a number of these units to address the needs of these prisoners confirms the importance of this initiatives, although the criteria for admission to a specialist unit need to be clearly defined and implemented; otherwise this becomes 'an unreliable public policy' (Wangmo et al., 2018).

High dependency unit, Rimutaka prison, New Zealand

The implementation of the High Dependency Unit (HDU) was a joint collaborative project with the Ministry of Health and the Department of Corrections (Brown, 2015; Brooke, 2018). The HDU is a 30-bedded unit for male prisoners, with complex health needs, including dementia, who require support with their activities of daily living. The majority of residents are over the age of 70; those with cognitive impairment or dementia are identified by prison staff because of a change in their behaviour, which has become disruptive or unusual. When admitted to the HDU, prisoners are screened for dementia and placed on a care plan. The care plans are regularly reviewed by the District Health Board through a Needs Assessment and Service Coordination (NASC) assessment. Prisoners on the HDU are supported by healthcare staff 24 hours a day, with one registered nurse and two to three healthcare assistants (HCAs).

Two prison officers remain on the unit and hold the keys to the patients' cells. The registered nurses, HCAs and prison officers work solely in the HDU and do not rotate with other staff within the prison. When prisoners are admitted to the HDU, they became recognised as patients.

The HDU includes two large day rooms, with access to an outside area; a laundry area; and a clinical room. The cells were contained in two corridors from either side of the day rooms. Each corridor contained two cells which were larger in size to support the use of hoists; however, all cells had hospital beds, shower and toilet. The day rooms contained televisions and tables where patients came together for their meals, complete puzzles and play card games. The day rooms were also used to hold weekly visits by animals including dogs, cats, a llama and pigs. The patients on HDU had complex health needs including restricted mobility. However, no family or friends were permitted to visit the HDU, so patients had to be transferred to the visitor area to receive any visitors, although this was supported by the HDU's own minibus. All the prisoners were considered patients once admitted to this unit but remained detained as prisoners, although few challenges of the rules or aggressive outbreaks were reported.

The Special Needs Program for Inmate-Patients with Dementia, USA

The adaptation of the physical environment to support the Special Needs Program for Inmate-Patients with Dementia (SNPID) has already been discussed earlier in this chapter. The interventions of this programme are implemented Monday to Friday, every week of the year (Hodel and Sanchez, 2012). Prisoners with dementia in this programme are supported by two nursing staff, a psychologist and three prisoners; alongside the custody staff nursing staff provided 24-hour care. Staff and prisoners received six months and 12 months respectively of training, which included causes and clinical presentation of dementia, effective communication and managing and identifying triggers for behaviours that challenge. Prisoners with dementia received individual interventions, such as pocket-sized flashcard to support each prisoner with their stressors, which included a pictorial presentation of their stressor on one side and how to appropriately address this stressor on the revise side. All prisoners with dementia were provided with recreational activities and group events during the day, and mornings would begin with an explanation of the day's activities, such as sensory stimulation or reminiscence, followed by a walk around the exercise yard. A preliminary evaluation of the programmes suggests a reduction in behaviours that challenge and agitation in prisoners with dementia (Hodel, 2009).

3 Purposive initiatives

Purposive initiatives that include meaningful or purposeful activities have been commenced to support older prisoners and those with dementia. These initiatives range from arts and crafts, music, social activities and light work (Brooke and Rybacka, 2020a; Wilkinson and Caulfield, 2017). These initiatives also significantly differ in the initiation, implementation, delivery and support, as some initiatives are provided by the prison, others by external agencies both charitable and limited companies and others by volunteers. Four of these different approaches will be described. However, there are many more examples in the literature, although a common thread is that all of these different approaches have been either anecdotally or qualitatively explored to demonstrate a positive impact on supporting older prisoners and those with dementia. Therefore, there is an element of caution before implementing such initiatives.

Two initiatives have been implemented in one prison in the South West of England, to support older prisoners and those with dementia. For the purpose of anonymity of participant's quotes, these initiatives have been called the Social Task Group and Purposive Activity Group (Brooke and Rybacka, 2020a).

Social Task Group

The Social Task Group was an initiative implemented by the prison to support prisoners over the age of 55, who no longer attended work. One prison officer is permanently rotated to support these older prisoners, both mornings and afternoons Monday through Friday. This initiative used a designated space that was solely used for this purpose, which included a number of converted cells for different arts and crafts, such as painting bird houses, alongside more practical work such as repairing wheelchairs for the Red Cross or packing breakfast bags. In total, ten cells were continuously occupied with various activities. All activities were prisoner led, and all prisoners were able to complete these activities independently, with approximately 30 prisoners attending each session. The designated space also included a large common room, which facilitated older prisoners to meet and socialise with tea and toast and was also used to show films and deliver talks from external visitors. Finally, the designated space was connected to an outside space that prisoners had permanent access to, although this was a concrete yard. Two prisoners attending this group recognised the importance of this initiative to support them through their prison sentence with other older prisoners:

> I find it (attending this group) interesting and you have the social aspect, they are all friendly and all sorts of odd bods. I am enjoying it, it is prison life you have got to do what you have got to do. I don't see it as being banged up as it isn't like that here (attending this group) they are all alright here, making cake and that, you drift along.

Purposive Activity Group

The Purposive Activity Group was an initiative led by education and delivered by one member of the education staff on the ground floor of a wing, which was designated for older prisoners with mobility difficulties. The initiative was implemented four mornings and afternoons each week and involved arts and crafts with problem-solving elements, as well a pop quizzes and discussions. One afternoon a week activities were held in the gym to encourage physical activity, which included games such as skittles and hula hoop. The older prisoners within this group required one-to-one or small-group supervision to engage and be supported through these activities; therefore this group was attended by only six to ten prisoners. A prisoner recognised the benefit of attending this group, as it enabled him to be out of his cell and socialise and provided him with something to do:

> This group is really good, because if we didn't do this during the week we would be locked up and we would have nothing to do, and on this course we do a bit of painting and making things, and we do a bit of answering questions, write some stories and things, and it is good to get out you know and be amongst others.

Good Vibrations Gamelan project

The Good Vibrations project is led by a charity and involves Gamelan music from Indonesia, which is played on bronze percussion instruments (Wilkinson and Caulfield, 2017). The weeklong project involves the learning of music, dance and shadow puppetry, with participants learning to improvise and compose their own pieces to perform at the end of the project to an audience. Previously, qualitative evaluations of the project when implemented with younger prisoners found a medication effect, which supported prisoners to manage their emotions, and a sense of motivation and achievement, alongside supporting communication and listening skills (Caulfield et al., 2016). Although these themes emerged from qualitative evaluations with older prisoners, there was also an emphasis on the accessibility of the project which was paramount because of their different levels of mobility, and it provided them with something meaningful to do and the ability to think about life beyond prison. The only negative element regarding this project was the one-off nature of attending and the project only lasted one week.

Art workshop

This is one initiative implemented for aging women prisoners and was a series of six art expression workshops, which was led by a group of volunteers who were social workers, marriage and family therapists, with no prison staff present during any of the workshops. The six expression workshops included an introduction, name embellishment, left-handed day, my first home, white-paper sculpture and an interactive group model project. This initiative was found to be supportive to aging women prisoners as it allowed them to dream, feel connected with fellow prisoners, who had a mutual understanding and therefore could release their feelings in an unselfish way (Hongo et al., 2015). The benefit of this low-cost initiative, which relied on volunteers, was that it encouraged older women prisoners to connect and support each other.

Summary

The prevalence of dementia in prison settings has been estimated, with a minimum of less than 1 per cent of the prison adult population to nearly 19 per cent of the prison population. A current issue with an accurate understanding of the breadth of dementia in prison is the lack of an appropriate cognitive screening tool, which would be sensitive within this environment. A screening tool has been developed in the USA, but it is unclear if this has been validated or is appropriate for other prison regimes around the world. The care and support of both older prisoners and those with dementia is hampered in many prisons, due to the physical environment of Victorian prisons, This is beginning to change with refurbishments and the building of new prisons. Four specific elements have been identified to improve the support and care for older prisoners and those with dementia, which include changes to the environment, education for prison staff, meaningful engagement and a collaborative approach. Specific initiatives were discussed, such as peer support including the Gold Coats and the Buddy Support Worker, specific units and the implementation of purposive initiatives.

References

Baidawi, S., Turner, S., Trotter, C., Browning, C., Collier, P., O'Connor, D., Sheehan, R. (2011). Older prisoners: a challenge for Australian corrections. *Trends and Issues*, 426.

Bedard, R., Metzger, L., Williams, B. (2016). Aging prisoners: on introduction to geriatric health-care, challenges in correctional facilities. *International Review of the Red Cross*, 98(903): 917–939.

Belluck, P. (2012). Dementia behind bars makes caregivers of killers: inmates change from predators to protectors, aid system stressed by growing demands. *New York Times*, February 25. Available from: www.nytimes.com/2012/02/26/health/dealing-with-dementia-among-aging-criminals.html [Accessed on: 15 May 2020].

Berry, S., David, T., Harvey, D., Hendersen, S., Hughes, B., Law, S., Hongo, A. (2016). *The Gold Goats: An Exceptional Standard of Care*. Washington, DC: Amazon Great Britain.

Brooke, J.M. (2018). Supporting prisoners with cognitive impairment and dementia in the prison setting. *2018 Winston Churchill Memorial Trust Fellowship* (unpublished report).

Brooke, J.M., Diaz-Gil, A., Jackson, D. (2020). The impact of dementia in the prison setting: a systematic review. *Dementia*, 19(5): 1509–1531.

Brooke, J.M., Jackson, D. (2019). An exploration of the support provided by prison staff, education, health and social care professionals, and prisoners for prisoners with dementia. *The Journal of Forensic Psychiatry and Psychology*, 30(5): 807–823.

Brooke, J.M., Kirk, M. (2014). Advance-care planning for people with dementia. *British Journal of Community Nursing*, 19(10): 422–427.

Brooke, J.M., Rybacka, M. (2020a). Exploration of two prison initiatives to support older prisoner's social needs: an inductive phenomenological study of prisoners lived experience. *International Journal of Prison Health*, DOI: 10.1108/IJPH-03-2020-0016.

Brooke, J.M., Rybacka, M. (2020b). Development of a dementia education workshop for prison staff, prisoners, health and social care professionals. *Journal of Correctional Healthcare*, DOI: 10.1177/1078345820916444.

Brown, J.A. (2015). *Living with Dementia in Prison. The Winston Churchill Memorial Trust of Australia*. Available from: www.churchilltrust.com.au/media/fellows/Brown_J_2015_Living_with_dementia_in_prison.pdf [Accessed on: 15 May 2020].

Byers, A.L., Yaffe, K. (2011). Depression and risk of developing dementia. *Nature Reviews Neurology*, 7: 323–331.

Care Act 2014 c 23. Her Majesty's Stationery Office: London.

Carpenter, B., Dave, J. (2004). Disclosing dementia diagnosis: a review of opinion and practice, and a proposed research agenda. *Gerontologist*, 44(2): 149–158.

Caulfield, L.S., Wilkinson, D.J., Wilson, D. (2016). Exploring alternative terrain in the rehabilitation and treatment of offenders: findings from a prison-based music project. *Journal of Offender Rehabilitation*, 55(6): 396–418.

Caverley, S.J. (2006). Older mentally ill inmates: a descriptive study. *Journal of Correctional Health Care*, 12: 262–268.

Cloyes, K.G., Rosenkranz, S.J., Wold, D., Berry, P.H., Supiano, K.P. (2014). To be truly alive: motivation among prison inmates hospice volunteers and the transformative process of end-of-life peer care services. *American Journal of Hospice and Palliative Medicine*, 31(7): 735–748.

Combalbert, N., Pennequin, V., Ferrand, C., Armand, M., Anselme, M., Geffray, B. (2018). Cognitive impairment, self-perceived health and quality of life of older prisoners. *Criminal Behaviour and Mental Health*, 28(1): 36–49.

Combalbert, N., Pennequin, V., Ferrand, C., Vandevyvere, R., Armand, M., Geffray, B. (2016). Mental disorders and cognitive impairment in ageing offenders. *The Journal of Forensic Psychiatry and Psychology*, 27: 853–866.

Corrada, M.M., Brookmeyer, R., Paganini-Hill, A., Berlau, D., Kawas, C. (2010). Dementia incidence continues to increase with age in the oldest old: the 90+ study. *Annals of Neurology*, 67(1): 114–121.

Corrada, M.M., Hayden, K.M., Paganini-Hill, A., Bullain, S.S., DeMoss, J., Aguirre, C., Brookmeyer, R., Kawas, C.H. (2017). Age of onset of hypertension and risk of dementia in the oldest-old: the 90+ study. *Alzheimer's & Dementia*, 13(2): 103–110.

de Vleminck, A., Pardon, K., Beernaert, K., et al. (2014). Barriers to advanced care planning in cancer, heart failure and dementia patients: a focus group study on general practitioners' views and experiences. *PLoS One*, 9(1): e84905.

Dementia Action Alliance (2018). *Dementia Friendly Physical Environment Checklist*. Available from: www.dementiaaction.org.uk/assets/0000/4336/dementia_friendly_environments_checklist.pdf [Accessed on: 15 May 2020].

Dening, K.H., Jones, L, Sampson, E.L. (2011). Advance care planning for people with dementia: a review. *International Psychogeriatrics*, 23(10): 1535–1551.

Di Lorito, C., Vollm, B., Dening, T. (2018). Psychiatric disorders among older prisoners: a systematic review and comparison study against older people in the community. *Aging and Mental Health*, 22(1): 1–10.

Dickinson, D., Bamford, C., Exley, C., Emmett, C., Hughes, J., Robinson, L. (2013). Planning for tomorrow whilst living for today: the views of people with dementia and their families on advance care planning. *International Psychogeriatrics*, 25(12): 2011–2021.

Dillon, G., Vinter, L.P., Winder, B., Finch, L. (2018). 'The guy might not even be able to remember why he's here and what he is in prison for and why he's locked in': residents and prison staff experiences of living and working with people with dementia who are serving prison sentences for a sexual offence. *Psychology, Crime and Law*, 25(5): 440–457.

du Toit, S.H.J., McGrath, M. (2018). Dementia in prisons – enabling better care practices for those ageing in correctional facilities. *British Journal of Occupational Therapy*, 81(8): 460–462.

Fazel, S., Hope, T., O'Donnell, I., Jacoby, R. (2001). Hidden psychiatric morbidity in elderly prisoners. *British Journal of Psychiatry*, 179: 535–539.

Folstein, M., Folstein, S., McHugh, P. (1975). "Mini-mental state": a practical method for grading the cognitive state of patients for the clinician. *Journal of Psychiatric Research*, 12: 189–198.

Fratiglioni, L., Paillard-Borg, S., Winblad, B. (2004). An active and socially integrated lifestyle in late life might protect against dementia. *The Lancet Neurology*, 3(6): 343–353.

Gaster, B., Larson, E.B., Curtis, J.R. (2017). Advance directives for dementia: meeting a unique challenge. *JAMA*, 318(22): 2175–2176.

Gaston, S. (2018). Vulnerable prisoners: dementia and the impact on prisoners, staff and the correctional setting. *Collegian*, 25: 241–246.

Grant, A. (1999). *Elderly Inmates: Issues for Australia. Trends & Issues in Crime and Criminal Justice No. 115.* Canberra: Australian Institute of Criminology.

Grassian, S. (2008). Neuropsychiatric effects of solitary confinement. In A.E. Ojeda (Ed.) *The Trauma of Psychological Torture* (pp. 113–126). Westport, CT: Praeger, Greenwood Publishing Group.

Gray, T. (2018). North-east prison – officers given dementia training sessions. *The Press and Journal*. Available from: www.pressandjournal.co.uk/fp/news/north-east/1527557/prison-officers-given-dementia-training-sessions/ [Accessed on: 15 May 2020].

Harding, M. (2015). Advance care planning for people with dementia. *Primary Care (General Practice)*. Available from: https://patient.info/doctor/advance-care-planning [Accessed on: 15 May 2020].

Harrison, M. (2006). True grit: an innovative program for elderly inmates. *Corrections Today*, 68(7): 46–49.

Hayes, A.J., Burns, A., Turnbull, P., Shaw, J. (2012). The health and social needs of older male prisoners. *International Journal of Geriatric Psychiatry*, 27: 1155–1162.

Hodel, B. (2009). *Improving Dementia? First Results of Therapeutic Interventions for Inmate-Patients Experiencing Dementia.* Paper presented at the Festival of Scholars, Thousand Oaks, CA.

Hodel, B., Sanchez, H.G. (2012). The special needs program for inmate-patients with dementia (SNPID): a psychosocial program provided in the prison system. *Dementia*, 12(5): 54–660.

Hongo, A., Katz, A., Valenti, K.G. (2015). Art: Trauma to therapy for aging female prisoners. *Traumatology*, 21(3): 201–207.

Human Rights Watch (2012). *Old Behind Bars: The Aging Prison Population in the United States.* Human Rights Watch. Available from: www.hrw.org/sites/default/files/reports/usprisons0112webwcover_0.pdf [Accessed on: 15 May 2020].

Kingston, P., Le Mesurier, N., Yorston, G., Wardle, S., Heath, L. (2011). Psychiatric morbidity in older prisoners: unrecognized and undertreated. *International Psychogeriatrics*, 23: 1354–1360.

Kitwood, T. (1997). *Dementia Reconsidered: The Person Comes First.* Berkshire: Open University Press.

Koenig, H.G., Johnson, S., Bellard, J., Denker, M., Fenlon, R. (1995). Depression and anxiety disorder among older male inmates at a federal correctional facility. *Psychiatric Services*, 46: 399–401.

Kopera-Frye, K., Harrison, M.T., Iribarne, J., Dampsey, E., Adams, M., Grabreck, T., McMullen, T., Peak, K., McCown, W.G., Harrison, W.O. (2013). Veterans aging in place behind bars: a structured living program that works. *Psychological Services*, 10(1): 79–86.

Kouyoumdjian, F.G., Andreev, E.M., Borschmann, R., Kinner, S.A., McConnon, A. (2017). Do people who experience incarceration age more quickly? Exploratory analyses using retrospective cohort data on mortality from Ontario, Canada. *PLoS One*, DOI: 10.1371/journal.pone.0175837.

Lee, C., Haggith, A., Mann, N., Kuhn, I., Carter, F., Eden, B., van Bortel, T. (2016). Older prisoners and the care act 2014: an examination of the policy, practice and models of social care delivery. *Prison Service Journal*, 224: 35–41.

LoGiudice, D., Smith, K., Thomas, J., Lautenschlager, N.T., Almeida, O.P., . . . Flicker, L. (2006). Kimberley indigenous cognitive assessment tool (KICA): development of a cognitive assessment tool for older indigenous Australians. *International Psychogeriatrics*, 18: 269–280.

Maschi, T., Kwak, J., Ko, E., Morrissey, B. (2012). Forget me not: dementia in prison. *The Gerontologist*, 52(4): 441–451.

Masters, J.L., Magnuson, T.M., Bayer, B.L., Potter, J.F., Falkowski, P.P. (2016). Preparing corrections staff for the future: results of a 2-day training about aging inmates. *Journal of Correctional Health Care*, 22(2): 118–128.

McCrudden, K., Sindano, N. (2016). *Prison Inreach: Dementia Support Provision*. Available from: www.londonscn.nhs.uk/wp-content/uploads/2017/03/dem-prisons-1503171.pdf [Accessed on: 15 May 2020].

Mental Capacity Act 2005 c 9. Her Majesty's Stationery Office: London.

Ministry of Justice (2017). *Deaths in Prison Custody 1978 to 2018*. Available from: www.gov.uk/government/statistics/safety-in-custody-quarterly-update-to-march-2018 [Accessed on: 15 May 2020].

Moll, A. (2013). *Losing Track of Time, Dementia and the Aging Prison Populations; Treatment, Challenges and Examples of Good Practice*. Mental Health Foundation. Available from: www.mentalhealth.org.uk/sites/default/files/losing-track-of-time-2013.pdf [Accessed on: 15 May 2020].

Murdoch, N., Morris, P., Holmes, C. (2008). Depression in elderly life sentence prisoners. *International Journal of Geriatric Psychiatry*, 23: 957–962.

O'Hara, K., Forsyth, K., Senior, J., Stevenson, C., Hayes, A., Challis, D., Shaw, J. (2015). 'Social services will not touch us with a barge pole': social care provision for older prisoners. *The Journal of Forensic Psychiatry and Psychology*, 26(2): 275–281.

Ojo, O., Brooke, J. (2015). Evaluating the association between diabetes, cognitive decline and dementia. *International Journal of Environment Research and Public Health*, 12: 8281–8294.

Patterson, K., Newman, C., Doona, K. (2016). Improving the care of older persons in Australian prisons using the policy Delphi method. *Dementia*, 15(5): 1219–1233.

Poppe, M., Burleigh, S., Banerjee, S. (2013). Qualitative evaluation of advance care planning in early dementia (ACP-ED). *PLoS One*, 8(4): e60412.

Porteri, C. (2018). Advance directives as a tool to respect patients, values and preferences: discussions on the case of Alzheimer's disease. *BMC Medical Ethics*, 19: 9.

Prison and Probation Ombudsman (2013). *Learning from PPO Investigation, End of Life Care*. Available from: https://s3-eu-west-2.amazonaws.com/ppo-prod-storage-1g9rkhjhkjmgw/uploads/2014/07/Learning_from_PPO_investigations_-_End_of_life_care_final_web.pdf [Accessed on: 15 May 2020].

Prison and Probation Ombudsman (2016). *Learning Lesson Bulletin. Fatal Incidents Investigations*. Issue 11. Dementia. Available from: www.ppo.gov.uk/app/uploads/2016/07/PPO-Learning-Lessons-Bulletins_fatal-incident-investigations_issue-11_Dementia_WEB_Final.pdf [Accessed on: 15 May 2020].

Prison Service Instruction (2015). *External Prison Movement 33/2015*. Available from: www.justice.gov.uk/offenders/psis/prison-service-instructions-2015 [Accessed on: 15 May 2015].

Prison Service Instruction (2016). *Adult Social Care PSI 03/2016*. Available from: www.justice.gov.uk/offenders/psis/prison-service-instructions-2016 [Accessed on: 15 May 2020].

Regan, J.J., Alderson, A., Regan, W.M. (2002). Psychiatric disorders in aging prisoners. *Clinical Gerontologist*, 26: 117–124.

Reitz, C., den Heijer, T., van Dejin, C., Hofman, A., Breteler, M.M.B. (2007). Relation between smoking and risk of dementia and Alzheimer's disease. *Neurology*, 69(10): 998–1005.

Resettlement and Care of Older ex-Offenders (RECOOP) (2019). *The Care Act 2014 and The Buddy Support Worker Training Programme*. Available from: www.recoop.org.uk/dbfiles/pages/151/Buddy-Support-Worker-Leaflet.pdf [Accessed on: 15 May 2020].

Robinson, L., Dickinson, C., Bamford, C., Clark, A., Hughes, J., Exley, C. (2013). A qualitative study: professionals' experiences of advance care planning in dementia and palliative care, 'a good idea in theory but. . . '. *Palliative Medicine*, 27(5): 401–408.

Ruthirakuhan, M., Luedke, A.C., Tam, A., Goel, A., Kurji, A., Garcia, A. (2012). Use of physical and intellectual activities and socialization in the management of cognitive decline of aging and in dementia: a review. *Journal of Aging Research*, 2012: 384875.

Schmidhuber, M., Haeupler, S., Marinova-Schmidt, V., Frewer, A., Kolominsky-Rabas, P.L. (2017). Advance directives as support of autonomy for persons with dementia? A pilot study among persons with dementia and their informal caregivers. *Dementia and Geriatric Cognitive Disorders*, 7: 328–338.

Sharupski, K.A., Gross, A., Schrack, J.A., Deal, J.A., Eber, G.B. (2018). The health of American's aging prison population. *Epidemiologic Reviews*, 40(1): 157–165.

Shepherd, S.M., Ogloff, J.R.P., Shea, D., Pfeifer, J.E., Paradies, Y. (2017). Shepherd aboriginal prisoners and cognitive impairment: the impact of dual disadvantage on Social and emotional wellbeing. *Journal of Intellectual Disability Research*, 61(4): 385–397.

Social Services and Well-being Act (Wales) 2014 anaw 4. Her Majesty's Stationery Office: London.

South, J., Bagnall, A.M., Hulme, C., Woodhall, J., Longo, R., Dixey, R., Kinsella, K., Raine, G., Vinall-Collier, K., Wright, J. (2014). A systematic review of the effectiveness and cost-effectiveness of peer-based interventions to maintain and improve offender health in prison settings. *Health Services Delivery Research*, 2: 35.

Stewart, W. (2018). What does the implementation of peer care training in a UK prison reveal about peer engagement in peer caregiving? *Journal of Forensic Nursing*, 14(1): 18–26.

Stewart, W., Edmond, N. (2017). Prisoner peer caregiving: a literature review. *Nursing Standard*, 31(32): 44–51.

Treacy, S., Haggith, A., Wickramasinghe, N.D., van Bortel, T. (2019). Dementia-friendly prisons: a mixed methods evaluation of the application of dementia-friendly community principles to two prisons in England. *BMJ Open*, 19: e030087.

Van der Steen, J.T., van Soest-Poortvliet, M.C., Hallie-Heierman, M., et al. (2014). Factors associated with initiation of advance care planning in dementia: a systematic review. *Journal of Alzheimer's Disease*, 40(3): 743–757.

Wangmo, T., Handtke, V., Bretschneider, W., Elger, B.S. (2018). Improving the health of older prisoners: nutrition and exercise in correctional institutions. *Journal of Correctional Health Care*, 24(4): 52–364.

Wangmo, T., Meyer, A.H., Bretschneider, W., Handtke, V., Kressig, R.W., Gravier, B., Bula, C., Elger, B.S. (2015). Ageing prisoners' disease burden: is being old a better predictor than time serviced in prison? *Gerontology*, 61: 116–123.

Wilkinson, D.J., Caulfield, L.S. (2017). The perceived benefits of an arts project for health and wellbeing of older offenders. *Europe's Journal of Psychology*, 31(1): 16–27.

Williams, B.A., Goodwin, M.D., Baillargeon, J., Ahalt, C., Walter, L.C. (2012). Addressing the aging crisis in U.S. Criminal justice healthcare. *Journal of American Geriatric Society*, 60(6): 1150–1156.

Williams, B.A., Lindquist, K., Hill, T., Baillargeon, J., Mellow, J., Greifinger, R., Walter, L.C. (2009). Caregiving behind bars: correctional officer reports of disability in geriatric prisoners. *Journal of American Geriatric Society*, 57: 1286–1292.

Wilson, J., Barboza, S. (2010). The looming challenge of dementia in prison. *Correct Care*, 24(2): 10–13.

Wolters, F.J., Segufa, R.A., Darweesh, S.K.L., Bos, D., Ikram, M.A., Sabayan, B., Hofman, A., Sedaghat, S. (2018). Coronary heart disease, heart failure, and the risk of dementia: a systematic review and meta-analysis. *Alzheimer's & Dementia*, 14(11): 1493–1504.

5 Human rights in prison and dementia

Joanne Brooke

Human rights in prison

This section will provide a historical overview of the development of human rights for all individuals and those serving time in prison. It will commence with an introduction of the International Bill of Human Rights established by the United Nations (UN) and includes the:

- Universal Declaration of Human Rights (1948)
- International Covenant in Civil and Political Rights (1966)
- International Covenant on Economic, Social and Cultural Rights (1966).

The UN International Convention on Elimination of All Forms of Racial Discrimination (1965) and Convention on the Elimination of All Forms of Discrimination Against Women (1979) will be briefly discussed. The Declaration on the Rights of Disabled Persons (1975) and the Convention on the Rights of Persons with Disabilities (2006) will also be discussed in the following section alongside people with dementia.

However, the main discussion of this section will focus on the development of human rights for prisoners in the UN Standard Minimum Rules for the Treatment of Prisoners [The Nelson Mandela Rules] (2015). Article 10 of the covenant and Rule 1 of the standard states a person deprived of their liberty shall be treated with humanity and dignity, and both focus on prisons as reform and rehabilitation institutions. The last element of reform and rehabilitation is an important element to introduce as there is a need to adapt this approach to support aging prisoners with poor health including dementia, to ensure they are treated with humanity and dignity.

The United Nations (UN) is a global organisation founded following the Second World War and the atrocities that occurred. Originally, 51 countries were members of the UN; today there are 193 members. The UN was founded to support the continuation of world peace; enable friendly relations among nations and collaborations to improve the lives of those in need, including fighting hunger, disease and illiteracy; and finally to promote nations' respect for each other's freedoms and rights.

Before the introduction of Declarations and Covenants within the International Bill of Human Rights, a brief definition of the terms applied to different documents follows:

Declaration: a document stating agreed standards but which is not legally binding.
Convention: a document stating agreed standards, which is legally binding; this term is used synonymously with treaty or covenant.
Covenant: a document stating agreed standards, which is legally binding; this term is used synonymously with treaty or convention.

Universal Declaration of Human Rights (1948)

The Universal Declaration of Human Rights (UDHRs) was adopted by the United Nations General Assembly in 1948. The development of the UDHRs occurred through the initiation of a commissioned body within the UN, which represented global communities, including Australia, Belgium, Chile, China, Egypt, France, India, Iran, Lebanon, Panama, the Philippines, the UK, the US, USSR, Uruguay and Yugoslavia. The UDHRs was the first document to state that every human being is equally entitled to rights and freedom and has become the gold standard by which human rights are measured. The document has been translated into more than 360 languages and is the most translated document in the world (United Nations, 2015).

The General Assembly proclaims the Universal Declaration of Human Rights is

a common standard of achievement for all peoples and all nations, to the end that every individual and every organ of society, keeping this Declaration constantly in mind, shall strive by teaching and education to promote respect for these rights and freedoms and by progressive measures, national and international, to secure their universal and effective recognition and observance, both among the peoples of Member States themselves and among the peoples of territories under their jurisdiction.

(United Nations, 2015, p. 3)

The Articles of the Universal Declaration of Human Rights (1948) are briefly described in Table 5.1.

International Covenant on Civil and Political Rights (1966)

The International Covenant on Civil and Political Rights (1966) came into force in 1976, contains six discrete parts and is sometimes referred to as the first generation of rights. Part one, which only includes Article 1, emphasises the freedom and rights of individuals to choose and develop their own political,

Table 5.1 The Articles of the Universal Declaration of Human Rights (1948)

Article	Definition
Article 1	*We are all born free and equal* All human beings are born free and equal in dignity and rights and should respect and act towards each other with dignity.
Article 2	*Freedom from Discrimination* All human beings have the rights and freedoms documented within the Universal Declaration of Human Rights without distinction or discrimination against ethnicity, colour, gender, language, religion, political, national or social origin, property, birth or any other status, including the country or territory a person belongs.
Article 3	*Right to Life* All human beings have the right to life, freedom and security.
Article 4	*Freedom from Slavery* No human being will be held in slavery; slavery and the slave trade is banned.
Article 5	*Freedom from Torture* No human being will be tortured or receive punishment that is cruel, inhuman or degrading.
Article 6	*Right to Recognition Before the Law* All human beings have the right to recognition as a person before the law in every land.
Article 7	*Rights to Equality Before the Law* All human beings are equal before the law and are entitled to equal protection without discrimination.
Article 8	*Right to Remedy* All human beings have the support and protection of the law when fundamental rights are violated.
Article 9	*Freedom from Arbitrary Detention* No human being shall be arrested, detained or exiled due to an individual's random choice or whim.
Article 10	Right to a Fair Trial All human beings are entitled to a fair and public trial by an independent and impartial judge and jury.
Article 11	*Presumption of Innocence and International Crimes* All human beings have the right to be presumed innocent until proven guilty in a court of law with adequate defence. No human being will be found guilty of an offence that was not an offence at the time when it was committed.
Article 12	*Right to Privacy* All human beings have the right to privacy, including their families, correspondence, honour and reputation.
Article 13	*Freedom of Movement* All human beings have the right to freedom of movement both within their country and to leave and return to their own country.
Article 14	*Right to Asylum* All human beings have the right to seek and obtain asylum from persecution, unless this is due to non-political crimes completed by the individual, which contradict the Universal Declaration of Human Rights.
Article 15	*Right to Nationality* All human beings have the right to nationality, not be deprived of or denied to change their nationality.

(Continued)

Table 5.1 (Continued)

Article	Definition
Article 16	*Right to Marry and to Found a Family*
	Both men and women of legal age may marry without limitations due to race, nationality or religion, and have a family.
	Both parties will only enter into marriage once given free and full consent.
Article 17	*Right to Own Property*
	All human beings have the right to own property, alone or with others, and shall not be deprived of this property.
Article 18	*Freedom of Religion and Belief*
	All human beings have the right to freedom of thought, including religion and other beliefs, engaging with this privately or within a community, and the freedom to change religion and other beliefs.
Article 19	*Freedom of Opinion and Expression*
	All human beings have the right to hold and express opinions, and the right to share these through media sources.
Article 20	*Freedom of Assembly and Association*
	All human beings have the freedom and right to form peaceful groups and meetings, and nobody shall be forced to belong to a group or attend meetings.
Article 21	*A Short Course in Democracy*
	All human beings have the right to take part in the government of their country, either directly or through representation; a government which is elected periodically through genuine elections with secret voting.
Article 22	*Right to Social Security*
	All human beings should be supported to develop to their best ability through access to work, cultural activity and social security and have the freedom to develop their personality.
Article 23	*Right to Work*
	All human beings have the right to work, to choose their occupation, and work in favourable conditions, without the risk of unemployment.
	All human beings have the right to equal pay for the same work.
	All human beings have the right and freedom to join a trade union to protect their own interests.
Article 24	*Right to Rest and Leisure*
	All human beings have the right to rest and leisure time, with limitations of working hours and holidays with pay.
Article 25	*Right to Adequate Standard of Living*
	All human beings have the right to live with adequate resources to maintain their health and well-being, including sufficient food, clothing, housing and healthcare, with the right of support due to unemployment, sickness, disability, bereavement, retirement or the inability to work.
	All expectant mothers and their babies are entitled to specific care and support. All children when born have the same rights.
Article 26	*Right to Education*
	All human beings have the right to education, for children primary education should be free, higher education should be available for all who pass the necessary requirements.
	Education at all levels will support the development of individuals and provide an understanding of human rights, including the promotion of tolerance and friendship between the differences of people, countries and nations, such as religious beliefs.
	All parents have a choice of the type of education their children receive.

Article	Definition
Article 27	Right to Cultural, Artistic and Scientific Life
	All human beings have the right and freedom to become involved in cultural, arts and scientific communities and enjoy the benefits.
	All human beings have the right for their artistic or scientific work protected and benefit from them.
Article 28	Right to a Free and Fair World
	All human beings have the right to a social and peaceful world and the rights and freedoms stated within the Declaration of Human Rights.
Article 29	Duty to Your Community
	All human beings have a duty to their community, which provides them with the ability to develop to their full potential.
	The only limitations on all human beings' rights and freedoms will be to ensure these rights and freedoms for others, to maintain morals and laws in a democratic society.
Article 30	Rights Are Inalienable
	No human being, government or collective should act or plan to act in any way that would destroy the rights and freedoms of the Universal Declaration of Human Rights.

Adapted from United Nations (2015) and information from the United Nations Human Rights Office of the High Commissioner web page (accessed 2020).

economic, social and cultural goals and to dispose of their income as they wish. Part two, Articles 2–5, describes the necessary legislation to support and rectify any violation of the rights of this covenant. The only time these rights can be restricted is during a public national or international emergency. Part three, Articles 6–27, contains the rights of this covenant, which are drawn from the Universal Declaration of Human Rights (1948). Part four, Articles 28–45, describes the development, reporting and monitoring of this covenant by the Human Rights Committee. Part five, the next two Articles, acknowledges that these rights do not interfere with the rights of people to freely engage and use their national resources. Part six, the final Articles, governs the enforcement, ratification and amendments to the covenant.

International Covenant on Economic, Social and Cultural Rights (1966)

The International Covenant on Economic, Social and Cultural Rights (1966) came into force in 1976 and is structured similar to the International Covenant on Civil and Political Rights (1966), with five discrete parts. Part one, which only includes Article 1, emphasises the freedom and rights of individuals to choose and develop their own political, economic, social and cultural goals and to dispose of their income as they wish. Part two, Articles 2–5, applies the concept of progressive realisation, the process of identifying the needs of disadvantaged populations and working towards rectifying these situations, such as equal access to healthcare. Part three, Articles 6–15, is also drawn from the Universal Declaration of Human Rights (1948), although it focuses on working environments, social security, parental leave, adequate standard of living, education and freedom to be involved in cultural life. Part four, Articles 16–25, describes the development, reporting and monitoring of this covenant by the UN Committee on Economic, Social and Cultural Rights. Part five, the final Articles, governs the enforcement, ratification and amendments to the covenant.

International Convention on the Elimination of All Forms of Racial Discrimination (1965)

The International Convention on the Elimination of All Forms of Racial Discrimination (1965) followed the Declaration on the Granting of Independence to Colonial Countries and Peoples (1960) and the Elimination of All Forms of Racisim (1963). The convention commits the members of the UN to actively address and eliminate racial discrimination and promote understanding within and across all races, which is monitored by the Committee on the Elimination of Racial Discrimination. The convention is divided into three parts, with 18 Articles. The first part of the convention defines racism, followed by the prevention of discrimination, condemnation of apartheid, prohibition of incitement and promotion of tolerance. The remaining two parts of the convention identify national dispute resolution mechanisms, including individual complaints mechanisms and the role of the Committee on the Elimination of Racial Discrimination.

Convention on the Elimination of All Forms of Discrimination Against Women (1979)

The Convention on the Elimination of All Forms of Discrimination Against Women (1979), came into force in 1981 and has since been ratified by 189 states. This was the first international law forbidding discrimination against women and enforcing all governments to work towards and advance the equality of women. The convention is divided into six discrete parts, with 30 Articles. Part 1 begins with the definition of the discrimination against women and the legal obligation of each state which adopts this convention. Discrimination against women is described as:

> any distinction, exclusion or restriction made on the basis of sex which has the effect or purpose of impairing or nullifying the recognition, enjoyment or exercise by women, irrespective of their marital status, on a basis of equality of men and women, of human rights and fundamental freedoms in the political, economic, social, cultural, civil or any other field.
>
> (UN, 1979)

The second part encompasses women's rights and representation in political and public life and entitlement to a nationality. The third part encompasses women's rights with regard to education, employment, health and economic and social benefits. The fourth part encompasses changes to law, and women's rights concerning marriage and family life. The fifth and sixth parts describe the monitoring, reporting and administration of this convention by the Committee on the Elimination of Discrimination against Women.

UN Standard Minimum Rules for the Treatment of Prisoners [The Nelson Mandela Rules] (2015)

The Standard Minimum Rules for the Treatment of Prisoners were first introduced in 1955 and remained unchanged for 60 years. In 2011, governments around the world agreed to review these rules and update them to reflect the changes in both criminal justice and human rights declarations and conventions (as described earlier). In 2014, the new rules, which updated eight areas of guidance, were adopted by the UN as the Mandela Rules (2015). The 122 rules are divided into two parts: part one explores the general management of prisons and is applicable to all prisoners, containing Rules 1–85. Whereas, guidance in part two is divided into sections specifically for prisoners under sentence (Rules 86–108), prisoners with mental disabilities and/or health conditions (Rules 109–110), prisoners under arrest or awaiting trial (Rules 111–120), civil prisoners (Rule 121) and finally people arrested or detained without charge (Rule 122). The following section will provide a brief overview of part one of the Mandela Rules, although a number of rules are not discussed, which include information to and complaints by prisoners, retention of prisoner's property, notification, investigations, removal of prisoners, institutional personnel and internal and external inspections. This will be followed by an overview of section A of part two of the Mandela Rules, which includes the rules for prisoners under sentence. Section B of part two, which is specifically relevant to prisoners with mental disabilities and/or health conditions, will then be explored.

Part one: rules of general application

Basic principles: the basic principles focus on the human rights of all prisoners and acknowledge their value as human beings and therefore to be treated with dignity. The application of all of the 122 rules are to be implemented impartially with no discrimination, and to support the equity of those with physical, mental or other disabilities. The basic principles commence with the rule to prevent torture, and other cruel, inhuman or degrading treatment or punishment of any prisoner. Therefore, prison regimes must not further affect prisoners' suffering, as prisoners have been deprived of their liberties to protect society and reduce recidivism. All prisons have a responsibility to support prisoners to reintegrate into society by providing education, vocational training, work and other forms of assistance to meet their needs.

Prisoner file management: these rules inform the information that needs to be obtained on the admission of a prisoner to prison, which is required to be stored within a standard prisoner file management system that ensures confidentiality and does not allow unauthorised access or modification of information. The information stored includes legal information regarding the prisoners' crime and sentence, but also their gender identity, family details and emergency contacts.

Separation categories and accommodation: prisoners will be separated according to their sex, age and criminal record. All prisoners shall be provided with an individual cell or room, except in extraordinary circumstances, such as temporary overcrowding. The implementation of dormitories needs regular supervision at night. All accommodation shall have enough natural light, ventilation and adequate access to be properly maintained and clean washing and toilet facilities.

Personal hygiene, clothing and bedding and food: all prisoners have a personal responsibility to keep themselves clean, and therefore the necessary toiletries will be provided, including shaving equipment for men. Also, all clothing worn needs to be clean and appropriate; if clothing is provided by the prison, this must not be degrading or humiliating. All prisoners will be provided with bedding in accordance with local or national standards. All prisoners will be provided with nutritional food at appropriate times throughout the day, although drinking water should always be available.

Exercise and sport: all prisoners are entitled to an hour a day of suitable exercise in the open air, weather permitting. Facilities to support physical and recreational training must be provided.

Healthcare services: all prisoners will be seen and examined by a healthcare professional on admission to prison. Healthcare for prisoners is to be provided at the same standard available in the community, which is the responsibility of the state. Healthcare provision should be organised to ensure the continuity of treatment and care, including treatment for infectious diseases and drug dependencies. All prisons need to provide healthcare services within the prison to support both the physical and mental health of prisoners. Emergency medical treatment shall be provided and if necessary, prisoners will be transferred to a specialised hospital. These decisions cannot be overruled or ignored by the prison administration. Healthcare professionals shall have daily access to all prisoners who are acutely unwell. The relationship between healthcare professionals and prisoners is governed by the same ethical and professional standards as those applied to these relationships in the community. Healthcare professionals are responsible to report any concerns regarding prisoner's health that may be due to imprisonment or they suspect/become aware of any signs of torture or other cruel, inhuman or degrading treatment or punishment.

Restriction, discipline, sanctions: safe custody and security of the prison shall be maintained with no more restriction than is necessary. Only competent authorities are allowed to identify conduct that is a disciplinary offence, and the types and duration of sanctions that can be imposed, including separation from the general prison population, such as solitary confinement, isolation and segregation. However, prisoners will only be sanctioned in a fair and due process and never twice for the same offence. A prisoner's mental health or developmental disability must be considered during this process. Restrictions, discipline and sanctions shall never amount to torture or other cruel, inhuman or degrading treatment or punishment. This includes restraints or restrictions on family visits. Healthcare professionals and other prisoners should have no role in the decision or implementation of disciplinary sanctions. Healthcare professionals have a responsibility to report any negative consequences of a sanction of a prisoner's physical and mental health.

Instruments of restraint and searches of prisoners and cells: restraints that are degrading and painful are prohibited. Instruments of restraint should only be applied when authorised by law to prevent escape during a transfer, a court appearance or prevent injury to themselves or others; in the latter cases, a healthcare professional will immediately be alerted. When a prisoner is restrained, the least intrusive method will be used, for the least length of time possible. All staff who apply restraints will be appropriately trained. Searches of prison cells should only occur within international law and conducted in a respectful manner providing dignity and privacy to the prisoner. Intrusive searches of prisoners will only be completed when absolutely necessary, and then by a healthcare professional or a member of staff who has been trained by a healthcare professional.

Contact with the outside world: prisoners shall be allowed to communicate at regular interviews with friends and family members through letters, phone calls or emails, or by receiving visits. Wherever possible, prisoners will be located in a prison close to their home. All prisoners shall have an adequate opportunity to meet and consult confidentially with their legal advisor. Foreign nationals shall be provided with reasonable access to communicate with diplomatic representation of their state.

Books and religion: every prison shall have a library stocked with both recreational and instructional books, and prisoners will be encouraged to use it. Prisons shall appoint a qualified religious representative, who will provide regular services and pastoral visits; when there are numerous prisoners with the same religion, this person should be permanent and on a full-time basis. This rule recognises the need for every prisoner to meet their religious needs, as far as this is possible.

Part two: prisoners under sentence

Guiding principles: the guiding principles include the responsibilities of the prison administration to begin the process of reintegration to society, which can commence with prisoners assisting staff with tasks to support social rehabilitation. All prisoners shall have a social worker who is charged with the responsibility of supporting family relations and contact with relevant agencies.

Prisoners in this stage of their sentence may be moved to an open prison, as they do not require the same degree of security.

Treatment: the sense of treatment in this rule is to enable prisoners to become law abiding and self-supporting on release and to encourage their self-respect and develop a sense of responsibility. To achieve these ends, all appropriate means shall be used, such as religious, education and vocational training, guidance on employment, physical and mental health development, whilst taking into account their social and criminal history.

Classification and individualisation and privileges: classification within this rule refers to the separation of prisoners who may have a bad influence on their peers or the division of prisoners depending on their treatment and rehabilitation needs. The development of individualised treatment plans for each prisoner is required that specifically addresses their individual needs, capacities and dispositions. In each prison, privileges will depend on the class of the prisoner and the different treatments being undertaken. Privileges are to encourage a sense of responsibility, good conduct, alongside interest and cooperation in their treatment.

Work: all prisoners will have the opportunity to work, subject to their physical and mental fitness. Prison work will not be afflictive in nature or personally benefit prisoners or prison staff. However, the work should increase the prisoner's employability on release, such as the development of a trade. Where possible, the prisoners will be able to choose the work they undertake. Prisoners will be remunerated for their work and shall be allowed to spend part of their earnings, send a part home to their families and the remaining will be given to the prisoner on release.

Education and recreation: education will be compulsory for prisoners who are illiterate. For other prisoners, education will be integrated with the educational system of the country, so on release from prison, the prisoner can continue their studies. The maintenance of relationships between prisoners and their families shall be supported, alongside contact with agencies outside of the prison to support reintegration. Recreational and cultural activities shall also be provided in all prisons to support prisoners' physical and mental health.

Human rights in dementia

This section will commence with an introduction of UN declarations and conventions for people with disabilities, although these do not specifically include those with dementia. It will then discuss why a human rights-based approach to dementia care is essential and provide an early example of how the rights of people with dementia have been considered, with the discussion of the Charter of Rights for People with Dementia and their Carers in Scotland (Cross-Party Group in Scottish Parliament, 2009). This will be followed by the World Health Organization's (2015) focus on ensuring a human rights-based approach for people with dementia and a discussion of the rhetoric to reality of this approach. Lastly, it will present a contemporary concept of human rights of people with dementia, and the elements of PANEL: Participation in decisions that affect their human rights; Accountability of those responsible for the respect, protection and fulfilment of human rights; Non-discrimination; Empowerment to know their rights and how to claim them; and Legality, that is all decisions occur within the legal standards of human rights.

Declaration on the Rights of Disabled Persons (1975)

The Declaration on the Rights of Disabled Persons (1975) is a call for national and international action for people classified as disabled and contains 13 rights. The declaration commences with a definition of a disabled person, which is 'any person unable to ensure by himself or herself, wholly or partly, the necessities of a normal individual and/or social life, as a result of deficiencies, congenital or not, in his/her physical or mental capabilities.' From this definition of a disabled person, it is clear this can be applied to people with dementia, as their disease progresses, although this has not been recognised or agreed nationally or internationally. The declaration states all disabled persons should enjoy the rights set out within it without any form of distinctions or discrimination. The rights for people who are disabled include respect of their human rights; equal civil and political rights as others; the right to support to empower them to be as self-reliant as possible; right to medical, psychological and functional treatment, including rehabilitation and vocational training; right to economic and social security; right to live with their families and engage in all social, creative and recreational activities; right to be protected against all exploitation; right to access legal aid; and the right to be consulted in all matters pertaining to their rights as disabled persons.

UN Convention on the Rights of Persons with Disabilities (2006)

The UN Convention on the Rights of a Person with Disabilities contains 50 Articles and commences with the purpose and definition of this convention, followed by Articles 4 to 32, which are the rights of the person with disabilities, and lastly Articles 33 to 50, the governance of the convention by the Committee on the Rights of Persons with Disabilities, and the formal government ratification process and that of amendments. The convention defines people with disabilities as 'those who have long-term physical, mental, intellectual or sensory impairments which in interaction with various barriers may hinder their full and effective participation in society on an equal basis with others.' The convention includes specific articles relating to women with disabilities, children with disabilities and aspects of awareness raising, accessibility, right to life, and equal recognition before the law, including access to justice. More explicitly, the rights include the freedom from torture, or cruel or inhuman or degrading treatment or punishment; freedom from exploitation, violence and abuse; and freedom of expression and opinion, and access to information. The rights then include the right to liberty of movement and nationality, to live independently and to be included in the community, ensuring respect for the person with disabilities privacy, including privacy of their home and their family, the right to appropriate and gold-standard education, healthcare, rehabilitation, work and employment, whilst supporting people with disabilities to participate in political and public life, as well as cultural life, recreation and leisure activities.

Dementia, rights, and the social model of disability: a new direction for policy and practice? (Mental Health Foundation, 2015)

The Mental Health Foundation (2015) in this document describes the social model of disability with regard to dementia, where people with dementia are at the centre of this model and their voices are heard, and they are recognised as equal citizens with rights. The social model of dementia includes the development of dementia-friendly communities and a human rights-based approach to dementia care, both of which are discussed later. The implementation of a social model requires changes at individual, institutional and systematic levels to evoke the changes necessary to support people with dementia. Until recently, dementia has not been recognised as a disability in policy, and in international law is still not recognised in this way. Simultaneously the human rights of people with dementia have not been a focus. The terminology of dementia as a disability does not focus on what the person cannot do, but rather, with changes in society, what a person with dementia can do. The following sections introduce the human rights-based approach to dementia care.

Human rights-based approach to dementia care

A human rights-based approach to dementia care is essential, as people with dementia are often denied their human rights and are at risk of mistreatment (Hansberry et al., 2005). A review of current literature suggests that people with dementia are at a higher risk of physical (11 per cent) and psychological (19 per cent) domestic abuse than people without dementia (McCausland et al., 2016). An example of care, which is against an individual's human right concerns the use of restraints, both physical and chemical. A study exploring restraints in care provided to nursing home residents with dementia in Europe identified 19.6 per cent and 68.2 per cent were restrained physically and chemically respectively, and more concerning 12.2 per cent were restrained both physically and chemically (Foebel et al., 2016). Another form of abuse that has been documented to be prevalent against people with dementia is that of financial abuse, both in the early and later stages of the disease, which is often hidden and avoids public scrutiny, leaving little to no protection for someone with dementia (Manthorpe et al., 2012; Dalley et al., 2017). Therefore, legislation alone is insufficient, and there is a need for a human rights-based approach to support and care for individuals with dementia.

Charter of Rights for People with Dementia and their Carers in Scotland (Cross-Party Group in Scottish Parliament, 2009)

The development of this charter involved members of the Scottish Parliament and organisations representing people with dementia, with an emphasis on ensuring the rights of people with dementia and those who sort them are recognised and supported. The charter adopted the approach of PANEL, which is recognised and endorsed by the UN. PANEL will be discussed in depth in the last section of this chapter, but briefly it involves:

- **P**articipation – all individuals should be included in decisions that may affect their human rights.
- **A**ccountability – all individuals have the right to respect, protection, and fulfilment of their human rights.
- **N**on-discrimination and equality – no individuals should be discriminated against and all individuals should be treated equally.
- **E**mpowerment – all individuals must be able to understand their human rights and know how to claim these rights.
- **L**egality – all decisions should occur through abiding by human rights legal standards and international laws.

The Charter of Rights for People with Dementia and their Carers in Scotland (2009) includes 15 rights under the headings of PANEL:

Participation includes how people with dementia can meaningfully participate in society. What is important here is meaningful, not tokenistic, participation. The element of participation also aligns with person-centred care: the person with dementia is at the centre of the decisions made about them. As stated by Dementia Alliance International, 'nothing about us without us.' Dementia Alliance International is a non-profit organisation run by people with a diagnosis of any type of dementia for people with any type of dementia. The rights of participation for people with dementia and their family members include:

1   accessible information to support them to participate in decisions that affect them;
2   live as independently as possible, with access to leisure, cultural and religious life;
3   participation in identifying and planning care to address their needs, including end-of-life care;
4   participation in the development and implementation of policies to support the human rights of people with dementia and their family members.

Accountability requires appropriate laws, policies and procedures to ensure the following rights are adhered to and appropriate mechanisms are in place when these human rights are violated or neglected. The rights include:

5   the rights of people with dementia to enjoy the fundamental free-doms embedded in human rights with respect, dignity and privacy;
6   organisations supporting and caring for people with dementia are accountable for their provision of respectful and dignified care which encompasses the human rights of the person with dementia.

Non-discrimination and equality enforce the need for all types of discrimi-nation, both direct and indirect, to be prohibited and prevented, especially for those who are most vulnerable. Discrimination towards a person with dementia can reduce their opportunities to participate in society, but also their development and growth (Woods, 2001). The right includes:

7   the right to be free from discrimination.

Empowerment involves the process of people both knowing and under-standing their rights and how to claim them and includes the rights of people with dementia to:

8   access appropriate care, which includes elements of rehabilitation;
9   help to support and maintain their independence, including physi-cal, mental, social and vocational abilities, which will enable them to be fully included in all aspects of life;
10   access to education and lifelong learning;
11   access to social and legal services to inform and enhance autonomy;
12   access to health and social care services provided by profession-als who are competent in providing dementia care from a human rights-based perspective.

Legality refers to the important fact that human rights are legally enforcea-ble through national and international human rights legislation. Regarding dementia, all policies, practice and research should be aligned with human rights legislation. This includes the rights for people with dementia to:

13   have their human rights respected, protected and fulfilled;
14   to information and participation in decision making and if their rights are not observed, to have access to a complaint and appeal process;
15   to the same civil and legal rights as individuals without dementia. If an individual lacks capacity for specific decisions, the principles of the Adults with Incapacity (Scotland) Act 2000 must be adhered to,

and all decisions must benefit the person, restrict their freedoms as least as possible, and respect their previous wishes and that of those who know them.

Ensuring a human rights-based approach for people living with dementia (World Health Organization, 2015)

The World Health Organization (WHO, 2015) acknowledges the need to ensure a human rights-based approach for people with dementia. This document applies the approach of PANEL and provides practical and implemented examples from around the world. These examples are going to be explored in more depth next.

Participation

In the UK, the Prime Minister's Challenge on Dementia (Department of Health, 2012) supported the initiative commenced by Alzheimer's Society, 'Dementia Friends'. The aim of this initiative was to create one million dementia friends across England and Wales, which was achieved in 2015. This has now increased to two and a half million in 2020. The Dementia Friends initiative is one of the largest initiatives to challenge people's perceptions of dementia at a population level, with the aim to change negative attitudes and the language applied to people with dementia. The initiative supports the participation of people with dementia in their community for longer, through raising awareness, and provides the general population with advice on how to support people with dementia to continue to participate in society. Anybody can become a dementia friend, by learning about dementia, through engaging with the Alzheimer's Society, to enable them to support people with dementia in their community. A central objective of being a dementia friend is the development of an inclusive community, where stigma, lack of understanding, loneliness and social exclusion are reduced.

The Dementia Friends initiative has been expanded to the development of dementia-friendly communities (DFCs), which is also supported by the Prime Minister's Challenge on Dementia and the Alzheimer's Society (2013). The ethos of creating DFC is to 'encourage everyone to share responsibility for ensuring that people with dementia feel understood, valued and able to contribute to their community'. The development of DFC includes the involvement of people with dementia and their families and friends and the wider community to address a number of important elements: challenge stigma and increase understanding; ensure community activities are accessible; acknowledge the potential of people with dementia; early diagnosis and post-diagnosis support; practical support to enable engagement in the community, perhaps a befriending service; relevant and practical community-based solutions; consistent and reliable travel options; an environment that is easy to navigate; respectful and responsive businesses and services, including training of staff. Many other organisations have become involved in DFCs such as Age UK, public services, churches, superstores, banks, schools and hospitals. Although this is a UK example, there are other examples, such as from the US and 'A tool kit for building dementia friendly communities' (Wisconsin Department of Health Services, 2015).

Accountability

In the UK, the accountability of NHS Trusts to provide competent and skilled care to support patients with dementia has been supported through organisational wide programmes of education and training, relevant documentation, staffing roles, and changes to the hospital environment. A common element of these programmes is that of mandatory dementia awareness training for all staff. Barbara's Story is one example that was widely implemented (Baillie et al., 2016). This approach included the development of an ethnodrama based on an older woman called Barbara, which aimed to emotionally engage staff through a series of films that showed Barbara's experience and perspectives of everyday healthcare. An element to support training is the implementation of supportive documentation, such as 'Getting to Know Me' (Elvish et al., 2014) and 'This is Me' developed by the Alzheimer's Society. Both of these documents aim to improve staff knowledge of the patient with dementia, with the provision of a card, which remains with the patient whilst in hospital. The card is completed by healthcare staff with the person with dementia and their families to support their care and understand their needs whilst in the hospital. Information includes likes and dislikes, such as favourite drinks and food, personal preferences regarding hygiene routines and taking medication, and interests, as well as television or radio preferences. The implementation of new staff roles has also occurred. One example is that of Dementia Champions within acute hospitals within Scotland to act as change agents, who with training and support developed action plans to improve the care of patients with dementia (Banks et al., 2014). Finally, the improvement of hospital environments has been supported by the development of a checklist created by the Kings Fund (2014), 'Is your ward dementia friendly? Environmental Assessment Tool', which focused on five important aspects of meaningful activity, legibility, orientation, wayfinding and familiarity.

Non-discrimination and equality

The support of non-discrimination for people with dementia has occurred through mass media advertising campaigns in many countries. An example provided by WHO (2015) is that of Brazil. The Alzheimer's Association in Brazil organised a nationwide television campaign to support and raise general awareness and education of the general population of dementia, with the aim of decreasing stigma. The campaign included a famous actress to engage with the viewers. Following the campaign, the numbers of calls to the Alzheimer's

Society helpline doubled. In the UK, nationwide television campaigns have been part of an awareness campaign, including more recently a television show 'The Great Canal Journeys', which featured a famous actress Prunella Scales and her husband. Prunella was diagnosed with dementia before the filming of these shows, which provide a true picture of the abilities of a person with dementia, and the enjoyment and memories of past events as the couple revisited a number of canal journeys they had completed when their family was young.

Empowerment

The ability of people with dementia to make decisions is often debated. However, a Norwegian study explored how people with dementia were able to participate in the decision-making process and the influence of their family members and healthcare professionals (Smebye et al., 2012). A number of different categories of decision-making processes were identified in people with moderate dementia, including pseudo-autonomous, delegated, shared, autonomous and non-involvement. Pseudo-autonomous decision making occurred when decision making was implicit rather than explicit and a lack of informed discussion occurred. Delegated decision making occurred when the person with dementia consciously deferred the decision-making responsibility to another person. Shared decision making was the most common type and involved informed discussions. Autonomous decision making mostly occurred when the person with dementia completed daily activities rather than major decisions. Lastly, non-involvement decision making occurred when the progression of the dementia was such that the person was no longer capable of being involved in the decision-making process. This study focused on the need to involve people with dementia in decision making and the need to recognise that people with dementia are capable of making decisions. Family members and health and social care professionals need to ensure the person with dementia has understood the decision to be made, which may include the restructuring or simplifying the information and providing cues to prompt memory and narrowing the range of choices (Smebye et al., 2012).

Legality

The World Health Organization (2015) includes the Charter of Rights for People with Dementia and their Carers in Scotland (Cross-Party Group in Scottish Parliament, 2009) as an example of a human rights-based approach for people with dementia. This has been further supported in Scotland with the development of their National Dementia Strategy (2017–2020) from this rights-based approach. The vision of the strategy clearly focuses on the human rights of people with dementia: 'a Scotland where people with dementia and those who care for them have access to timely, skilled and well-coordinated support from diagnosis to end of life which helps achieve the outcomes that matter to them'. The strategy contains 21 commitments, which build on previous strategies, but with three main components: the first is the commitment of timely, person-centred, consistent treatment and care for people with dementia and their family members, across all settings. The second commitment is to make further progress on the provision of support following diagnosis, and through the trajectory of the disease, with consideration of individual's needs and circumstances. Finally, the third component is a focus on responding to the increasing number of older people developing dementia in later life, often among the onset of other long-term conditions.

Therefore, it becomes clear that human rights-based approaches for people living with dementia need to be embedded in national dementia strategies. A number of countries have adopted this approach in the development of their national dementia strategies including Scotland (as discussed earlier), Norway and their Dementia Plan 2020, US and their National Plan to Address Alzheimer's Disease: 2016 Update, and Australia with their National Framework for Action on Dementia 2015–2019. Although human rights are embedded within these strategies, there is an emphasis on civil and political rights, rather than social rights, and an emphasis on the negative rather than positive rights, again with the exception of Scotland's National Dementia Strategy 2017–2020 (Cahill, 2018).

Human rights of prisoners with dementia

This section will draw on information provided in the two preceding sections of this chapter and develop thinking and recommendations to support people with dementia within a prison setting, as well as explore part two of the UN Standard Minimum Rules for the Treatment of Prisoners [The Nelson Mandela Rules] (2015), which explicitly refers to prisoners with mental disabilities and/or health conditions. The relevance and adaptation of the UN Convention of the Rights of Persons with Disabilities (2006) to support prisoners with dementia is an important and essential approach to enable the appropriate health and social care for these prisoners. The information provided and discussed in this section will be presented under each of the PANEL headings: Participation, Accountability, Non-discrimination, Empowerment and Legality.

Participation

Participation in prison activities such as vocational training, education, sport and social cultural activities has been recognised to support the reduction of recidivism and improve prisoner's self-worth and sense of well-being (Digennaro, 2010; Meek and Lewis, 2014; Peshers and Patterson, 2011). However, as explored in Chapter 4, initiatives within prison settings have focused on the rehabilitation and training of younger prisoners to support them on release and to find employment. This approach is not suitable or appropriate for older prisoners, or prisoners with dementia. In the UK, Her Majesty's Prison and

Probation Service commissioned the charity RECOOP (Resettlement and Care for Older ex-Offenders and Prisoners) to develop a good practice guide for working with older prisoners, which included prisoners with dementia. RECOOP (2017) identified the need to address a number of elements to support participation of older prisoners and those with dementia in workshops, education, purposeful activity and physical activity:

- Workshops: the importance of supporting prisoners to keep working past retirement if they so wished, with the option of part-time work, alongside active support, encouragement and motivation by prison staff for older prisoners and those with dementia to engage with workshops, where lighter and more accessible roles should be prioritised for older prisoners and those with dementia.
- Education: there was no age-specific education identified in prisons in the UK, although older prisoners' educational needs may be different from younger prisoners, as they may be interested in recreational learning to keep their minds occupied. Therefore, there was a need to develop education to support this specific need.
- Purposeful activity: in the prison setting, purposeful activity involves time out of the cell, education, work and physical activity, alongside behaviour programmes and visits from their legal team and family members. The recommendation from HM Inspectorate of Prisons is ten hours of purposeful activity on each weekday. However, RECOOP identified that older prisoners and those with dementia were spending longer locked in their cells. The most common reason identified was concerns regarding health, confidence in mixing with younger prisoners and a lack of interest in activities available, all of which needs to be addressed to enable participation of older prisoners and those with dementia.
- Physical activity: the most common forms of exercise within a prison is walking, gym exercise or work. A number of prisons in England and Wales have timetabled gym sessions for those over the age of 55 to allow older prisoners the confidence to attend.

Accountability

The provision of social care for older prisoners and those with dementia in England and Wales has been found to be lacking. HM Inspectorate of Prisons and the Care Quality Commission (CQC) (2018) found prisoners who are unable to care for themselves, mobilise independently or require support to participate in social activities are at a significant disadvantage. However, this has been addressed to a certain extent through legislation, as local authorities are now responsible and accountable for social care provided to prisoners in England and Wales. Although there remains no comprehensive national strategy for the provision of social care in prisons, the needs of older prisoners and those with dementia can be formerly assessed with the Older prisoner Health and Social Care Assessment and Plan (OHSCAP) (Walsh et al., 2014). Clear guidance has also been produced by other governing bodies, such as Public Health England (2017), which recognise the complexities and need for comprehensive social assessment of older prisoners. Unfortunately, inconsistency of comprehensive assessments of the social needs of older prisoners and those with dementia has led to inconsistent physical, emotional and social care support throughout a prison sentence and upon release (Di Lorito et al., 2018). Therefore, the provision of social care for older prisoners and those with dementia is still one that needs to be addressed and accountable authorities tasked with improving their provision of care.

Non-discrimination and equality

Non-discrimination of prisoners with dementia by prison staff requires the ability of staff to recognise and support prisoners with dementia, rather than reprimand behaviours that may challenge the prison regime, but of which the prisoner has no control (Carpenter and Dave, 2004). Prison staff as well as health and social care professionals working in prison settings have reported the difficulty of identifying signs of dementia because of other mental health conditions and reactions to illegal drugs (Gaston, 2018; Dillon et al., 2018). Dementia education has commenced in prison settings but tends to be limited to specific staff within specific dementia initiatives, or within the wider topic of supporting older prisoners (Hodel and Sanchez, 2012; Masters et al., 2016). In the UK, Dementia Friends sessions, as described earlier, have been delivered to staff and prisoners. However, prison staff require further information, such as recognising cognitive deterioration, communicating with a prisoner with dementia and supporting behaviours that may challenge the prison regime from a person-centred approach, to ensure non-discrimination towards these prisoners.

Education on dementia for prison staff and health and social care professionals needs to specifically focus on dementia in a prison setting and the unique challenges associated with this setting (Brooke and Rybacka, 2020). This approach can empower staff to support a prisoner with dementia, although prison culture, environment and regimes need to be simultaneously addressed by higher level government strategies and legislation. An example is the need to understand visual complications that arise from dementia, which include misinterpretation and identification, loss of depth perception and peripheral vision and shadowing (Alzheimer's Society, 2016). These visual difficulties can be supported through changes in the environment, such as good lighting, living space on the ground floor, removal of shiny floors and painting of walls, ceilings and doors so they are not the same colour (Kings Fund, 2013). These minor environment changes will help prisoners with dementia to be more independent, as these changes will aid them in understanding their surroundings. This is support through the implementation of DFC principles (described earlier in this chapter) in two prisons in England. Although successful, a lack of focus by the government on dementia in prison with appropriate funding and strategy meant this approach was not sustainable (Treacy et al., 2019).

Empowerment

A fundamental element of empowerment is being provided with all the information to make an informed decision. As discussed previously, the capacity of prisoners with dementia to make informed complex decisions is reduced as their disease progresses. Therefore, it is essential for prison, legal and health and social care staff to complete a functional assessment to determine if a patient is capable of making a specific decision. The ability to make an informed decision is always situation specific, and a prisoner with dementia make lack the capacity to make an informed choice regarding an upcoming appeal but can be supported to decide what they would like to eat. Refer to both Chapter 2 and Chapter 6 on a decision of capacity and in the UK, the Mental Capacity Act (2005).

Legality

The UN Standard Minimum Rules for the Treatment of Prisoners [The Nelson Mandela Rules] (2015) Part two, which relates to prisoners with mental disabilities and/or health conditions, clearly states that prisoners who are diagnosed with severe mental disabilities and/or health conditions should not be held within the prison setting if this further exacerbates their condition and should be transferred to mental health facilities, or facilities within the prison staffed by qualified healthcare professionals. This is an important consideration for prisoners with dementia, especially those who may develop dementia whilst in prison, as the onset is gradual and decline may occur over a number of years. Therefore, it is essential that prisoners with dementia have regular assessments of their cognitive abilities and their mental and physical health and how they are coping with the prison regime. Mental health considerations for people with dementia are an important aspect of their ongoing care due to the high prevalence of depression in this population (Kurling et al., 2018).

The Nelson Mandela Rules (2015) also state that prisoners should receive appropriate psychiatric assessment and treatment. Within the UK, a diagnosis of dementia occurs through a series of visits to a specialist memory service. A diagnosis of dementia involves a detailed medical history, a physical examination, blood tests, brain scans and an array of cognitive and neurological tests. In the Prison Service of England and Wales, there are currently no policies or guidelines to enable prisoners with cognitive decline to access these services. Following a diagnosis, dementia-specific treatment should commence within six weeks, alongside the development of a personal dementia care plan (NHS England, 2017). Once again, there is a lack of pathways in prison settings to support this care, which urgently needs to be addressed, as it is a legal right of all those with cognitive decline in prison.

Finally, prisoners with end-stage dementia should be considered for compassionate release, as this procedure typically allows prisoners to seek early release due to serious terminal, non-terminal and/or age-related health issues (Price, 2018). This currently has not occurred in the UK, perhaps because dementia has only recently been recognised as a terminal illness by those outside of the healthcare profession, and the trajectory of dementia for each individual is difficult to predict. In the UK, Early Release on Compassionate Grounds allows the secretary of state to release a prisoner on licence at any point in their sentence if 'exceptional circumstances' exist. These circumstances include 'terminal illness [where] death is likely to occur soon' and 'where the prisoner is bedridden or severely incapacitated' (HM Prison Service, 2005). These circumstances both clearly apply to a person with dementia as their disease progresses, and these rules need to be readdressed to consider and include those prisoners with dementia, as this is their right.

Summary

This chapter has explored the rights of all human beings, focused on the human rights of prisoners and then on the human rights of people with dementia. Human rights are appropriate for all human beings across all settings. However, different elements of human rights need to be explored and prioritised when considering the human rights of people in prison and those living with dementia. Within a prison setting, the importance of the UN Minimum Rules for the Treatment of Prisoners, the Nelson Mandela Rules cannot be over emphasized. Although there are no specific recommendations regarding prisoners with dementia, the rights of prisoners with mental disabilities are included. The human rights of people with dementia are now beginning to be recognized and addressed through policies, strategies and social models, which promote a human rights-based approach to support and care.

References

Alzheimer's Society (2013). *Building Dementia Friendly Communities: A Priority for Everyone.* Available from: https://actonalz.org/sites/default/files/documents/Dementia_friendly_communities_full_report.pdf [Accessed on: 21 May 2020].

Alzheimer's Society (2016). *Sight, Perception and Hallucinations in Dementia. Factsheet 527CP.* Available from: www.alzheimers.org.uk/sites/default/files/pdf/sight_perception_and_hallucinations_in_dementia.pdf [Accessed on: 21 May 2020].

Baillie, L., Sills, E., Thomas, N. (2016). Educating a health service workforce about dementia: a qualitative study. *Quality in Ageing and Older Adults*, 17(2): 119–130.

Banks, P., Waugh, A., Henderson, J., et al. (2014). Enriching the care of patients with dementia in acute settings? The Dementia Champions Programme in Scotland. *Dementia,* 13(6): 717–736.

Brooke, J.M., Rybacka, M. (2020). Development of a dementia education workshop for prison staff, prisoners, health and social care professionals. *Journal of Correctional Health,* DOI: 10.1177/1078345820916444.

Cahill, S. (2018). WHO's global action plan on the public health response to dementia: some challenges and opportunities. *Aging and Mental Health*, 24(2): 197–199.

Carpenter, B., Dave, J. (2004). Disclosing dementia diagnosis: a review of opinion and practice, and a proposed research agenda. *Gerontologist*, 44(2): 149–158.

Cross-Party Group in Scottish Parliament (2009). *Charter of Rights for People with Dementia and Their Carers in Scotland*. Available from: www.alzscot.org/sites/default/files/images/0000/2678/Charter_of_Rights.pdf [Accessed on: 21 May 2020].

Dalley, G., Gilhooly, M., Gilhooly, K., Harries, P., Levi, M. (2017). *Financial Abuse of People Lacking Mental Capacity. A Report to the Dawes Trust*. Available from: http://bura.brunel.ac.uk/handle/2438/15255 [Assessed on: 21 May 2020].

Department of Health (2012). *Prime Minister's Challenge on Dementia: Delivering Major Improvements in Dementia Care and Research by 2015*. Available from: https://assets.publishing.service.gov.uk/government/uploads/system/uploads/attachment_data/file/215101/dh_133176.pdf [Accessed on: 21 May 2020].

Di Lorito, C., Vollm, B., Dening, T. (2018). The individual experience of ageing prisoners: systematic review and meta-synthesis through a Good Lives Model framework. *International Journal of Geriatric Psychiatry*, 33(2): 252–262.

Digennaro, S. (2010). Playing in the jail: sport as psychosocial tool for inmates. *International Review on Sport and Violence*, 2: 4–24.

Dillon, G., Vinter, L.P., Winder, B., Finch, L. (2018). 'The guy might not even be able to remember why he's here and what he is in prison for and why he's locked in': residents and prison staff experiences of living and working with people with dementia who are serving prison sentences for a sexual offence. *Psychology, Crime and Law*, 25(5): 440–457.

Elvish, R., Burrow, S., Cawley, R., Harney, K., Graham, P., Pilling, M. (2014). 'Getting to know me': the development and evaluation of a training programme for enhancing skills in the care of people with dementia in general hospital settings. *Aging and Mental Health*, 18(4): 481–488.

Foebel, A.D., Onder, G., Finne-Soveri, H., Lukas, A., Denkinger, M.D., Carfi, A., Vertrano, D.L., Brandi, V., Bernabei, R., Liperoti, R. (2016). Physical restraint and antipsychotic medication use among nursing home residents with dementia. *JAMA*, 184: 9–14.

Gaston, S. (2018). Vulnerable prisoners: dementia and the impact on prisoners, staff and the correctional setting. *Collegian*, 25: 241–246.

Hansberry, M.R., Chen, E., Gorbien, J. (2005). Dementia and elder abuse. *Clinics in General Medicine*, 21(2): 315–332.

HM Inspectorate of Prisons and the Care Quality Commission (2018). *Care for Elderly Prisoners Is Inconsistent and the Lack of Planning for an Ageing Population Is a Serious Defect, Say Inspectors*. Available from: www.justiceinspectorates.gov.uk/hmiprisons/media/press-releases/2018/10/care-for-elderly-prisoners-is-inconsistent-and-the-lack-of-planning-for-an-ageing-population-is-a-serious-defect-say-inspectors/ [Accessed on: 21 May 2020].

HM Prison Service (2005). *Prison Service Order: 6000. Parole, Release and Recall*. Available from: www.justice.gov.uk/downloads/offenders/psipso/pso/pso-6000.pdf [Accessed on: 21 May 2020].

Hodel, B., Sanchez, H.G. (2012). The Special Needs Program for Inmate-patients with Dementia (SNPID): a psychosocial program provided in the prison system. *Dementia*, 12(5): 54–660.

The King's Fund (2013). *Improving the Patient Experience. Developing Supportive Design for People with Dementia. The King's Fund Enhancing the Healing Environment Programme 2009–2012*. Available from: www.kingsfund.org.uk/sites/files/kf/field/field_publication_file/

developing-supportive-design-for-people-with-dementia-kingsfund-jan13_0.pdf [Accessed on: 21 May 2020].

The King's Fund (2014). *Is Your Ward Dementia Friendly? EHE Environmental Assessment Tool.* 3rd edition. Available from: www.kingsfund.org.uk/sites/default/files/EHE-dementia-assessment-tool.pdf [Accessed on: 21 May 2020].

Kurling, J.K., Mathias, J.L., Ward, L. (2018). Prevalence of depression, anxiety and PTSD in people with dementia: a systematic review and meta-analysis. *Neuropsychology Review*, 28: 393–416.

Manthorpe, J., Samsi, K., Rapaport, J. (2012). Responding to the financial abuse of people with dementia: a qualitative study of safeguarding experiences in England. *International Psychogeriatrics*, 24(9): 1454–1464.

Masters, J.L., Magnuson, T.M., Bayer, B.L., Potter, J.F., Falkowski, P.P. (2016). Preparing corrections staff for the future: results of a 2-day training about aging inmates. *Journal of Correctional Health Care*, 22(2): 118–128.

McCausland, B., Knight, L., Page, L., Trevillian, K. (2016). A systematic review of the prevalence and odds of domestic abuse victimisation among people with dementia. *International Review of Psychiatry*, 5, DOI: 10.1080/09540261.2016.1215296.

Meek, R., Lewis, G. (2014). The impact of a sports initiative for young men in prison: staff and participant perspectives. *Journal of Sport and Social Issues*, 38(2): 95–123.

Mental Capacity Act 2005 c 9. Her Majesty's Stationery Office: London.

Mental Health Foundation (2015). *Dementia, Rights, and the Social Model of Disability. A New Direction for Policy and Practice?* Available from: www.mentalhealth.org.uk/sites/default/files/dementia-rights-policy-discussion.pdf [Accessed on: 21 May 2020].

NHS England (2017). *NHS England Dementia: Good Personalised Care and Support Planning Information for Primary Care Providers and Commissioners.* Available from: www.england.nhs.uk/wp-content/uploads/2020/02/FINAL-_Update_Dementia-Good-Care-Planning-.pdf [Accessed on: 21 May 2020].

Peshers, G., Patterson, G. (2011). Books open worlds for people behind bars. Library services in prison as exemplified by the Münster prison library, Germans library of the year 2007. *Library Trends*, 59(3): 520–543.

Price, M. (2018). *Families Against Mandatory Minimums, Everywhere and Nowhere: Compassionate Release in the States.* Available from: https://famm.org/wp-content/uploads/Exec-Summary-Report.pdf [Accessed on: 21 May 2020].

Public Health England (2017). *Health and Social Care Needs Assessments of the Older Prison Population.* London: PHE Publications.

RECOOP (2017). *Good Practice Guide: Working with Older Prisoners.* Available from: www.recoop.org.uk/dbfiles/pages/54/FINAL-Older-Prisoners-Good-Practice-Guide-2017.pdf [Accessed on: 21 May 2020].

Smebye, K.I., Kirkevold, M., Engedal, K. (2012). How do people with dementia participate in decision making related to health and daily care? A multi-case study. *BM Health Services Research*, 12: 241.

Treacy, S., Haggith, A., Wickramasinghe, N.D., van Bortel, T. (2019). Dementia-friendly prisons: a mixed methods evaluation of the application of dementia-friendly community principles to two prisons in England. *BMJ Open*, 9: e030087.

United Nations Department of Economic and Social Affairs. Convention on the Rights of Persons with Disabilities (2006). Available from: www.un.org/development/desa/disabilities/convention-on-the-rights-of-persons-with-disabilities.html [Accessed on: 21 May 2020].

United Nations Human Rights Office of the High Commissioner. 30 Articles of the Universal Declaration of Human Rights (1948). Available from: www.ohchr.org/en/News Events/Pages/DisplayNews.aspx?NewsID=23871&LangID=E [Accessed on: 21 May 2020].

United Nations Human Rights Office of the High Commissioner. Declaration on the Granting of Independence to Colonial Countries and Peoples (1960). www.ohchr.org/en/professionalinterest/pages/cescr.aspx [Accessed on: 21 May 2020].

United Nations Human Rights Office of the High Commissioner. Convention on the Elimination of All Forms of Discrimination Against Women (1979). Available from: www.ohchr.org/EN/ProfessionalInterest/Pages/CEDAW.aspx [Accessed on: 21 May 2020].

United Nations Human Rights Office of the High Commissioners. International Convention on the Elimination of All Forms of Racisim (1963). www.ohchr.org/en/profession alinterest/pages/cescr.aspx [Accessed on: 21 May 2020].

United Nations Human Rights Office of the High Commissioner. Declaration on the Rights of Disabled Persons (1975). Available from: www.ohchr.org/EN/Professional Interest/Pages/RightsOfDisabledPersons.aspx [Accessed on: 21 May 2020].

United Nations Human Rights Office of the High Commissioner. International Covenant on Civil and Political Rights (1966). Available from: www.ohchr.org/en/professional interest/pages/ccpr.aspx [Accessed on: 21 May 2020].

United Nations Human Rights Office of the High Commissioner. International Covenant on Economic, Social and Cultural Rights (1966). Available from: www.ohchr.org/en/ professionalinterest/pages/cescr.aspx [Accessed on: 21 May 2020].

United Nations Human Rights Office of the High Commissioner. International Convention on the Elimination of All Forms of Racial Discrimination (1965). Available from: www.ohchr.org/en/professionalinterest/pages/cerd.aspx [Accessed on: 21 May 2020].

United Nations Standard Minimum Rules for the Treatment of Prisoners [The Mandela Rules] (2015). Available from: https://cdn.penalreform.org/wp-content/uploads/1957/06/ENG.pdf [Accessed on: 21 May 2020].

Walsh, E., Forsyth, K., Senior, J., O'Hara, K., Shaw, J. (2014). Undertaking action research in prison: developing the Older prisoners Health and Social Care Assessment and Plan (OHSCAP). *Action Research*, 12(2): 136–150.

Wisconsin Department of Health Services, Alzheimer's Society, AARP Wisconsin and Dementia-Capable Wisconsin (2015). *A Tool Kit for Building Dementia Friendly Communities*. Available from: www.dhs.wisconsin.gov/publications/p01000-dfc.pdf [Accessed on: 21 May 2020].

Woods, R. (2001). Discovering the person with Alzheimer's disease: cognitive emotional and behavioural aspects. *Ageing and Mental Health*, 55(1): S7–S16.

World Health Organisation (WHO) (2015). *Ensuring a Human Rights-Based Approach for People Living with Dementia*. Available from: www.who.int/mental_health/neurology/dementia/dementia_thematicbrief_human_rights.pdf?ua=1 [Accessed on: 21 May 2020].

6 The ethics of healthcare in prison and dementia

Lydia Aston

Ethics of healthcare in prison

All healthcare is guided by the principles of medical ethics, and the first part of this section will explore these complex concepts, commencing with its four pillars: beneficence, non-maleficence, autonomy and justice (Beauchamp and Childress, 2001). The second part will explore the ethical and organisational provision of prison healthcare through the six principles of the United Nations (UN) Principles of Medical Ethics (1982) and the work of the Committee of Ministers of the Council of Europe (2006). The third part will discuss the disparity and difficulties between a theoretical approach to ethical healthcare and the practical provision of healthcare in prisons, exploring the challenges of confidentiality, informed consent and a duty of care (Lehtmets and Pont, 2014). The barriers to parity in healthcare in prison settings will then be examined through the UK government's health and social care reports (House of Commons Health and Social Care Committe, 2018) and the introduction of the European Committee for the Prevention of Torture and Inhuman or Degrading Treatment or Punishment (CPT) standards.

Medical ethics

Ethics is the philosophy and study of human conduct, which seeks to illuminate what is 'right' and 'correct' and 'wrong' and 'incorrect', and the general agreement between these considerations (Pont, 2006). Medical ethics has a focus on care and quality of life, alongside the definition of life. The debate of these concepts through history is long and complicated. However, Western medical ethics originates with the Hippocratic Oath in the fourth century BC, which informs the healthcare professional's ethical standards. Medical ethics is integrated into all aspects of care, and the ethical principles that healthcare professionals must adhere to have been contextualised into the four pillars of medical ethics: beneficence, non-maleficence, autonomy and justice (Beauchamp and Childress, 2001).

Beneficence

Beneficence with regard to healthcare is derived from humanism (Kinsinger, 2010). Simply, beneficence is the concept that all of humanity has the right to life. Thus, healthcare practitioners should enable the patient's health and well-being, providing good health to the best of their ability. An element of benefi-cence is doing good and seeking the 'right' thing for the patient, doing good for the patient. Therefore, clinical healthcare professionals and their practice should refrain from preventable practices that cause psychological, physical or moral harm (Munyaradzi, 2012). The provision of care requires a weighing of the pos-sibilities of good against the possible harms, and there is an obligation for health-care practitioners to provide care which benefits the patient (Beauchamp, 1989).

Non-maleficence

Healthcare professionals need to consider beneficence and non-maleficence simultaneously. As Gillon (1994) states, 'whenever we try to help others we inevitably risk harming them'. (p. 185). Healthcare professionals' decision to provide care must be formed through an understanding that minimal harm will occur to the patient and that the care is of benefit to them (Gillon, 1994). Therefore, healthcare professionals receive rigorous continual education and training to support them to avoid both intentional and unintentional harm. The provision of harm-free care where possible involves an autonomous, inter-active and transparent relationship of care between the healthcare practitioner and the patient, where decision making is shared between the involved parties (Sacristán et al., 2016).

Autonomy

Autonomy refers to the moral obligation to respect others' decisions when they have the capacity to deliberate and make their own decisions (Gillon, 1994), and the acknowledgement that people have the right to their own opinions, per-spectives, values and beliefs (Ethical Practice, 2020). In healthcare, patients have the right to make informed decisions to accept or reject care; therefore, medical information needs to be communicated in a clear, understandable way that is veracious. Respect for autonomy requires healthcare professionals to communi-cate with patients and engage with them in the decision-making process (Sacris-tán et al., 2016). Another prerequisite of respect for autonomy is confidentiality, which contributes to the patient's trust in healthcare professionals and thus ena-bles communication of sensitive topics to inform the decision-making process.

Justice

Justice is the fair distribution of care equitably between patients, with a moral obligation to act with impartial adjudication between competing claims (Alz-heimer Europe, 2010). Equity and equality are two principles of justice, which enable the fair distribution of healthcare provisions (Alperovitch et al., 2009). Equity is the provision of healthcare that people need, whilst equality is pro-viding the same healthcare to everyone, under the assumption that all people require the same level of healthcare. Equality sometimes negatively affects older people, those from ethnic minority backgrounds, or with a disability, or due to hospital budgets, which causes injustice (Alzheimer Europe, 2010). Gillon (1994) describes distributive justice as the fair distribution of scarce resources, rights-based justice as the respect for people's rights, and legal justice as the respect for morally acceptable laws. Justice, therefore, is the intrinsic quality of how a person is treated, rather than how they are treated in relation to others.

Organisational guidance of healthcare in prisons

On an international level, the principles for the ethical and organisational provision of prison healthcare are defined by the World Medical Association Declaration of Geneva (1948, latest version in 2006), the International Code of Medical Ethics (1949, latest revision in 2006), United Nations General Assembly resolution 37/194 (of 18 December 1982) and Recommendation No. R (1998) 7 of the Committee of Ministers of the Council of Europe of 8 April 1998. These provisions establish the rights of prisoners in terms of access to healthcare and guidelines for the organisational and administrative responsibilities of the prison system. The UN summarises six principles of medical ethics applied to the prison setting:

Principle 1: healthcare professionals caring for prisoners or those detained have a duty to provide them with support to both maintain their physical and mental health and treat all illness. The support and treatment must be of the same quality and standard as provided to those who are not imprisoned or detained.

Principle 2: healthcare professionals must not engage, actively or passively, in acts which constitute participation in incitement to or attempts to commit torture or other cruel, inhuman or degrading treatment or punishment.

Principle 3: healthcare professionals must not be involved in any professional relationship with prisoners or detainees, when the purpose is not solely to evaluate, protect or improve their physical and mental health.

Principle 4: healthcare professionals must not apply their knowledge and skills to assist in the interrogation of prisoners and detainees in a manner that may adversely affect the physical or mental health of prisoners or detainees, or participate in the certification of the fitness of prisoners or detainees for any form of treatment or punishment that may adversely affect their physical or mental health.

Principle 5: healthcare professionals must not participate in any procedure for restraining a prisoner or detainee unless such a procedure is determined in accordance with medical criteria as being necessary for the protection of the physical or mental health or safety of the prisoner or detainee, of his fellow prisoners or detainees, and presents no hazard to his physical or mental health.

Principle 6: there may be no derogation from the foregoing principles on any ground whatsoever, including public emergency.

Council of Europe's Health in Prisons Part III (2006)

The Council of Europe's Health in Prisons Part III (Council of Europe, 2006) emphasises the role of prison authorities to safeguard the health of all prisoners in their care, which is the foundation of healthcare in prisons. The provision of healthcare to prisoners should be equal to that provided to the community or nation of the location of the prison. Therefore, the ethical and medical organisation of prison healthcare should be in alignment with the administration of healthcare of the community or nation and provided to prisoners without discrimination of their legal situation, such as medical, surgical and psychiatric services. The conditions of the Council of Europe's Health in Prisons Part III (Council of Europe, 2006) and the practical implications have been discussed in Chapter 2.

Ethical healthcare in prison

The combination of principles of medical ethics and the organisation of ethical healthcare in prison settings raises three prominent issues (Pont, 2011). First, prisoners might question how they can trust a doctor who is employed by the prison. Second, doctors working in prison settings might struggle to: reconcile patient confidentiality, privacy and consent in the totalitarian prison environment; balance relationships between prisoners and prison staff; manage the competing pressures of maintaining professional independence whilst being employed by the prison administration; and provide optimal care in a low-resourced environment. Finally, prison staff may be concerned about the compatibility of medical confidentiality, patient consent and the doctor's professional independence with the security and safety of the prison, as well as how to warrant expensive medical care costs within already stretched prison budgets. Among these competing priorities and concerns it is essential for prison physicians to uphold medical ethics and ensure these ethics are understood and accepted by each stakeholder in the prison community (Penal Reform International, 2001; Pont, 2006).

These prominent issues include the importance of positive relationships: prisoners need to trust the prison doctor, prison doctors need to trust the prison staff and relationships must be transparent and reliable (Lehtmets and Pont, 2014). The ethical challenges of confidentiality, consent, duty of care, barriers to securing healthcare in prisons and dilemmas for prison doctors will now be discussed, with a focus on the UK prison systems.

Confidentiality

All prisoners have the right to seek healthcare in confidence, and this should not be screened by prison officers. Medical consultations and examinations should be performed as they are in non-prison settings, in a medical consultation room, which is private and confidential, one patient at a time, with no non-medical staff present. However, if an officer is required to be present during a consultation for security and safety reasons, the officer should distance themselves so as to not see or hear the discussion or examination (Pont, 2006). Medical records of prisoners are the responsibility of the healthcare professionals and only transferred within a multidisciplinary team through a secure data transfer system. Medical information regarding a prisoner cannot be disclosed to prison administration without the consent of the patient (Lehtmets and Pont, 2014). Any medication that is prescribed should be given to prisoners in either a pre-packed dosette box or directly from a nurse to the prisoner to maintain confidentiality. These principles seek to build and develop a trust within the prison healthcare setting.

Consent

Informed consent for a medical examination is a legal requirement for any examination, whether in prison or the community, a part of the ethical principle of autonomy and a human right. Thus, the prisoner must agree to any examinations or treatment offered. Difficulties with gaining informed consent in a prison setting may include a prisoner's abilities to read and write and understand the language used, not only medical terminology, but the language may be different from their native language (Lehtmets and Pont, 2014). An important role of prison doctors is to ensure that prisoners understand both examination processes and treatment options. This can be achieved by the doctor asking the prisoners to repeat back what they understand. However, implementation of informed consent may require adequate resources such as appropriate medical staff and the availability of translators (Pont, 2011).

Duty of care

International laws dictate that prisoners have the right to a safe and healthy environment (International Covenant on Civil and Political Rights, 1976; International Covenant on Economic, Social and Cultural Rights, 1976). The World Health Organization (WHO) states that governments have a special duty of care for those in places of detention and the recognition of human rights should be prioritised, including the right to health and healthcare (Gatherer et al., 2014). The right to health includes a preventative approach to healthcare, which should not be limited to curative or palliative medicine (Pont, 2006). A preventative approach to poor health is a public health priority; within prisons, this includes issues surrounding the inability to maintain a healthy lifestyle, such as the lack of opportunity to exercise and obtain a nutritional diet, alongside the need for substance rehabilitation and education and treatment for transmissible diseases (WHO, 2003; House of Commons Health and Social Care Committee, 2018). For prisoners who are terminally ill, arrangements should be made, wherever possible, for them to be transferred to the community or a prison hospital or hospice rather than their death to occur in a standard prison cell (Pont, 2006).

Dilemmas for prison doctors

The concept of professional independence for the healthcare professionals working in a prison setting can be challenging, as there is a need to balance their independence whilst working in and sometimes for a non-medical organisation, which is referred to as Dual Loyalty (Pont et al., 2012). This requires two layers of professional competence in possessing the medical skills and knowledge to be part of the healthcare team whilst also holding the specialist knowledge necessary to apply that within a prison setting. This is exemplified by the challenge of providing confidential care to patients whilst recognising the possible implications for the safety of the prison. The challenges faced by healthcare professionals in the prison setting are often underestimated, especially when consent is a requirement. A healthcare professional may note injuries from violence on a prisoner, which should be reported to the prison authorities, but this can only occur with the consent of the prisoner. If the prisoner refuses, the doctor faces a difficult decision as to support the best interests of the prisoner, as well as other inmates.

Support for healthcare professionals has been outlined by the European Committee for the Prevention of Torture and Inhuman or Degrading Treatment or Punishment (Council of Europe, 2006). The CPT consists of teams of impartial experts such as lawyers, medical doctors and specialists in prison or police matters (Council of Europe, 2020). European Union member states are governed by the CPT, which conducts visits to places of detention, such as prisons, immigration detention centres and social care homes to evaluate how people are being treated. The committee can interview anyone who is deprived of their freedom in private, gathering information of their experiences. Visits can be planned or unannounced, the latter particularly if the CPT considers it crucial to observe a serious situation (Council of Europe, 2020). However, the small number of visits carried out by the committee may indicate a small cumulative impact to influence the norms and culture within healthcare in prisons.

A focus of the CPT during their visits to prison healthcare services includes free access to a doctor for every prisoner, equivalence of care, patient consent and confidentiality, preventive health, humanitarian assistance, professional independence and professional competence (Council of Europe, 1993). Compliance with these principles promotes medical ethics in prison settings, yet significant non-compliance has resulted in a crisis being declared by the CPT, particularly highlighting the delay or absence of medical examinations, and the failure to adequately address instances of violence (Lehtmets and Pont, 2014). There is a need to continually strive to adhere to medical ethics in prison settings and to act within accordance of the CPT principles. Pont et al. (2015) discusses elements that still need to be addressed, which include promoting a prisoner's confidence in medical care in prison, providing healthcare professionals clear guidance to prevent misunderstandings and ensure the quality of healthcare within a prison and lastly, dealing with a situation of conflict.

The conflicting and competing demands of healthcare within a prison setting have been summarised by Pont (2011): confidentiality, privacy and consent versus security and safety; equivalence of medical care and free access to medical care versus lack of resources and overcrowding; professional independence versus employment by prison administrators; disease prevention versus pathogenicity of the prison; and prison health is public health versus lack of public support. Therefore, prison remains a challenging environment in which to manage healthcare in a way that aligns with medical ethics and prison administration priorities. The previous chapter has addressed and discussed the issue that the delivery of prison health is now the responsibility of state healthcare institutions and that healthcare professionals are less likely to be directly employed by the prison administration.

Ethics of healthcare for people with dementia

Ethics of healthcare for people with dementia concerns the morally right thing to do, and in the case of dementia, there may be many options and none unambiguously right. Therefore, discussions regarding care include judgements on the values of courses of action. Ethical concerns have been highlighted by family members of people with dementia regarding appropriate allocation of funds for healthcare, standards of care provided and people with dementia being enabled to be involved in this process (Pratt et al., 1987). The first part of this section will provide an overview of the spectrum of dementia-specific ethical issues (Strech et al., 2013). The second part will explore other ethical issues within healthcare for people with dementia, including advanced technology and the use of digital surveillance (Niemeijer et al., 2010). The last part will explore the provision of ethical healthcare for people with dementia through an ethical framework with six components, which was developed by the Nuffield Council on Bioethics (2009).

Dementia-specific ethical issues

The existence of disease-specific ethical issues in dementia care are recognised by international and national reports and clinical practice guidelines (Nuffield Council on Bioethics, 2009). Strech et al. (2013) conducted a systematic review to determine the full spectrum of ethical issues in dementia care. The review was purely descriptive as opposed to making judgements or recommendations on the practical relevance or value of each dementia-specific ethical issue. The review identified 56 disease-specific ethical issues within dementia care, which were aligned to the following seven major categories.

Diagnosis and medical indication

A prominent ethical issue was the need to provide adequate consideration of the complexity of diagnosing dementia, and the inclusion of the experiences and understanding of both the person with symptoms and their family members. This aspect included a consideration of the reasonableness of treatment indications, and the balance of communicating the potential effects of pharmaceutical treatment options to the person with dementia and their families, whilst managing a realistic sense of hope (Rabins and Black, 2010). A further prominent ethical issue identified was the need for healthcare professionals to have an adequate appreciation of the patient, which recognises the autonomy that should be given to a person living with dementia acknowledging them as a person and not a 'patient'. This extends to the perception of the quality of life of an individual living with dementia, as healthcare professionals often rate this lower than the person themselves.

Assessing patient decision-making competence

A prominent ethical issue was the ambiguity of understanding competence, which refers to the assessment of the competence of an individual to make an informed decision regarding their healthcare. Inadequacies in assessment of the capacity of people with dementia need to be addressed to ensure that the person's autonomy is respected and that they are provided every opportunity to make an informed decision (Hughes and Sabat, 2008).

Information and disclosure

An ethical issue concerns healthcare professionals respecting patient autonomy in the context of disclosure, which includes the need to seek the patient's permission and understand the amount of knowledge they wish to know regarding their health and the potential trajectory of short- and long-term outcomes of their dementia. Healthcare professionals need to respect the patient's autonomy, and by doing so only provide the level of information they wish to receive (Rabins, 2007). The information needs to be presented in a way and at a speed that is understandable, with possible repetition that allows the person with dementia to comprehend and assimilate the information being disclosed (Bavidge, 2006). A further ethical issue is the adequate involvement of family members, especially within the decision-making process. This is important as family members will need to make health decisions for the person with dementia, when their disease progresses and they lack both the capacity and the ability to communicate their decisions.

Decision making and consent

A number of ethical issues that need to be addressed were identified in the current process of involving people with dementia in the decision–making process, including inadequate involvement from the patient, insufficient conditions for nurturing decision-making capacity, disregarding the need for continuous relationship-building with the patient, and setting the time for decision-making processes. These issues relate to time, environing factors and relationships and the need to promote autonomy throughout the trajectory of the disease with a collaborative decision-making process (Oliver and Gee, 2009). However, eventually a person with dementia will need a surrogate to support decision making, which usually involves family members, who obtain a power of attorney. This process can be supported through the implementation of adequate living wills/advance directives to address the ethical challenges of advance planning for people with dementia (Brooke and Kirk, 2014).

Social and context-dependent aspects

Another ethical issued identified was the need to help relatives and clinical personnel and professional carers who are supporting a person with dementia. Ethical considerations of the impact of caring for a person with dementia are essential, as supporting a person with dementia involves more than just providing healthcare but the continuation or development of a therapeutic relationship, and the risk of burnout has been identified. A further ethical issue of the allocation of limited healthcare resources needs to be explored. It is essential to understand that the cost benefits of medical procedures and the delivery of care will benefit the individual with dementia and are in their best interests. These ethical considerations need to be explored to understand if the cost of resources informs clinical decisions, and if treatment is being withheld due to a diagnosis of dementia, which ultimately may have benefitted the person living with dementia.

Care process and process evaluation

An ethical issue within dementia care is the need for continuing assessment of potential benefits and harms, and the need to balance care between the commitment to not cause any harm, whilst being obliged to withdraw and withhold treatments that are causing harm. This deliberation in timing the shift in the nature of care, as well as considering a reasonable ceiling of care, poses complex ethical questions. Dementia is a terminal disease and end-of-life care will, at some point, involve the withdrawal of treatment. During the trajectory of the illness, it is important for family members caring for a relative with dementia to reflect on their experiences, and for healthcare professionals to recognise the complex difficulties family members face daily, which should be a point of regular discussions (Hughes, 2002).

Special situations for decision making

Situations that need specific ethical consideration in dementia care were identified by Strech et al. (2013) and include the ability to drive, sexual relationships, genetic testing, prescription of antibiotic and antipsychotic drugs, indication for brain imaging, covert medication administration, restraints, gastric feeding via a tube, end-of-life and palliative care and the use of monitoring techniques.

Advanced technology

An ethical issue that needs to be addressed within healthcare for people with dementia is the advanced technology and the use of digital surveillance (Niemeijer et al., 2010). Technology has emerged as a potential solution to a great number of pressures within the care sector, although ethical considerations need to be explored. Currently, a number of technological advancements could provide support to people living with dementia and their family members. These include:

- Smart homes, where physical human movement could trigger automatic lighting, automatic cut-offs for taps and cookers, and presence infrared (PIR) sensors, audio prompts, such as voices instructing or reminding the person with dementia to do something.
- Telecare and the use of monitors to support the physical health of a person living with dementia, which could include the provision of alerts to an appropriate person (such as a carer sleeping in a different room or a central monitoring service).
- Monitoring and tracking devices worn by the person with dementia, so that an alarm is sounded if the person moves away from a designated safe area, or so that the person's exact location can be identified if they get lost (Mental Welfare Commission for Scotland, 2007; Miskelly, 2005).
- Memory aids, such as audio recordings that provide the person with reminder messages or memory aids which stimulate a person's memory by automatically taking photographs of the events of the day.

The use of technology for people living with dementia could aid and provide an element of safety in assisting the person and support their family members. However, the use of such technologies gives rise to ethical debates regarding privacy and autonomy of the individual with dementia and the threat of those technologies replacing the relational aspects of care. The ethical deliberations on technology for people living with dementia focus on the moral acceptability of the way in which technology is used and its purposes (Niemeijer et al., 2010; Nuffield Council on Bioethics, 2009).

Ethically, there remains a lack of consensus on the use of surveillance and the contributions this can provide to the well-being and quality of life of the person living with dementia. Niemeijer et al. (2010) suggested that the following needs to be considered and balanced in using technologies to support people living with dementia: avoiding stigmatisation; enhancing freedom; respecting privacy, dignity and autonomy; and catering to the best interest of the person living with dementia. Whilst there are clear safeguarding benefits to surveillance being utilised within dementia care, the overall conclusions convey that devices should not be a substitute for person-centred care.

Ethical framework

The last part of this section will synthesise the ethical issues identified here and explore the provision of ethical healthcare for people with dementia, which has been supported by an ethical framework developed by the Nuffield Council on Bioethics (2009). The framework draws on the four pillars of medical ethics (Beauchamp and Childress, 2001) and has six components, which will now be explored.

Component 1: a case-based approach to ethical decisions

This component suggests a three-stage process for ethical decisions, which includes identifying and clarifying relevant factual considerations; interpreting and applying appropriate ethical values to those facts; and comparing with similar ethically relevant situations, exploring the similarities and differences between them. These stages support the idea that moral judgements should be based upon careful reflections of the contextual factors that are pertinent to the decision. Thus, decisions that are of a similar nature and that have already been made should be used as a comparison tool to assist in the decision in question. Consultations with legal frameworks and guidelines can be helpful, but the ambiguous nature of applying these in practice makes it difficult to be consistent and conclusive. Thus, the framework promotes a skills-and-knowledge approach to ethical decisions; for healthcare professionals, this requires continual education and forums in which experiences in practice can be shared and discussed. Information from these approaches to ethical dilemmas could then be shared with people with dementia and family members as a way of providing support during difficult decisions that may arise during dementia care.

Component 2: the nature of dementia

There are conflicting views on whether dementia constitutes a harm. This framework recognises that the disease is a harm, in that it is a degenerative brain disorder, which eventually has a negative impact on a person's quality of life. Dementia will also eventually affect a person's autonomy. There are three implications resulting from dementia being classified as a harm: first, research is imperative to discover a cure and improve the quality of life of people living with dementia. Second, reducing the rate of cognitive decline is important, whilst acknowledging the distress that this may cause a person living with dementia. Third, people living with dementia should be entitled to equal resource allocation for research, treatment and services as with any other terminal condition, such as cancer.

Component 3: quality of life in dementia

The third component argues that with compassionate and supportive care, it is possible for people with dementia to have a good quality of life throughout the illness experience. This framework recognises the experiences of living with dementia as a continuum, fluctuating between well-being and ill-being (Galvin and Todres, 2011; Todres and Galvin, 2006). A person living with the early stages of dementia can do so autonomously and achieve a good quality of life. A person's life is of value with or without cognitive impairment and the inability to reflect or be deliberative does not mean that life is not possible or that a good quality of life is not achievable. The quality of life of a person living in the middle- to end-stage dementia depends on family members and formal and informal carers, as well as at a broader societal level that recognises the value of providing care for people with dementia in supportive community environments.

Component 4: promoting interests in autonomy and well-being

This component promotes the continual strive for autonomy and well-being in people living with dementia. This involves continuing and enabling relationships that are meaningful to the person and giving the support they need in sustaining their sense of self and their values. Autonomy is not simply to be equated with the ability to make rational decisions. The promotion of autonomy and well-being needs to be considered separately for the person living with dementia, their family members and healthcare professionals. First, people with dementia need the freedom to make choices which are respected and endorsed, with the consideration of their best interests, as symptoms may preclude or limit effective decision making. In some cases, potentially harmful decisions may have to be negotiated or challenged by carers or professionals. However, this framework emphasises the need to support persons with dementia so that they can have the tools to express their sense of self rather than just being protected from harm. When the disease trajectory worsens, suitable advocates of the person with dementia need to be identified to actively support their autonomy. Encouraging and engaging with the person with dementia to make choices in the simple day-to-day life endorses autonomy, interweaves well-being and autonomy and places value on the person making the decision.

Second, family members provide most of the care for people with dementia living in the community. Therefore, it is essential that the interests of family members are considered as they may experience stressful encounters whilst supporting and caring for their relative. Support for family members or friends providing care should occur at a societal level and by healthcare professionals. The well-being and autonomy of the person with dementia is interwoven with that of family members; thus support for family members is likely to have a positive effect on the care they are providing (Hughes et al., 2002). The interests of family should be listened to attentively, particularly when conflicting issues are present in ethical decision making. Lastly, the support of healthcare professionals and social care workers working in dementia care is essential, including practical aspects of the work environment such as taking care of staffing levels, ensuring support through supervision and training and equipping staff with tools to ensure their care is holistic and beneficial.

Component 5: solidarity

The fifth component highlights the importance of a mutual responsibility to care for people with dementia at a societal level and within families. Solidarity becomes increasingly more significant to uphold especially when considering the prevalence of dementia and the continued risk of developing dementia in later life. Solidarity reinforces the need of recognition and accountability to de-stigmatise dementia within society, and society has a two-fold obligation to provide resources and support to people with dementia and their family members. Societally, the allocation of resources should lead to a supportive dementia care environment and aid in maintaining the well-being and autonomy of the person with dementia. People with dementia should be empowered and be given a voice where they need one, but they should also be included as a citizen in their own right and valued for their contribution (Houtepen and Meulen, 2000).

Component 6: recognising personhood

The recognition of personhood of people living with dementia emphasises the need to value them as they were before their diagnosis, which should continue throughout the course of their illness experience, regardless of cognitive and behavioural changes. For more information on personhood in dementia, refer to Chapter 3. In cases where a person's mood, behaviour and memory change profoundly, the person with dementia is still the same person, and this should guide policy and practice. The values and views a person with dementia had before the onset of their illness should assist the decision-making process when they no longer have the capacity.

Ethics of healthcare for prisoners with dementia

The last section of this chapter will synthesise the findings from the previous sections, including both the approach to healthcare in prisons and healthcare for people with dementia in the community, with the aim of constructing an ethical framework of healthcare for prisoners with dementia. The need for such a framework is overwhelming. First, almost two decades ago, Fazel et al. (2002) acknowledged the denial of access to appropriate healthcare for prisoners living with dementia, which represented a violation of their human rights. Second, as the overall prison population ages, and older prisoners have a high risk of developing dementia, the prevalence of dementia among prisoners is going to continue to increase (du Toit et al., 2019). Third, prisoners with dementia are the most vulnerable and neglected population within the prison (Maschi et al., 2012). In the UK, the need for an ethical framework for healthcare for prisoners with dementia has been identified by the Prison and Probation Ombudsman (2017) through the need to address the complex issues associated with prisoners with dementia. Therefore, the experience of living with dementia in the community, with family members present to support care, compared to experiences in prison requires careful scrutiny to ensure prisoners are being supported and cared for appropriately.

A tentative framework for ethical health and social care provision for prisoners with dementia has been developed from the previous two sections of this chapter. The ethical Health and Social Care Framework for the Provision for Prisoners with Dementia includes eight components: 1 screening, symptoms and diagnosis; 2 ethical decisions and patient decision-making competence; 3 information and disclosure; 4 recognising personhood; 5 family involvement; 6 care and evaluation of care; 7 environment; and 8 training for all staff.

1 Screening, symptoms and diagnosis

The identification of dementia in prison has been recognised as problematic, as some of the routines and rules within the prison regime could mask the onset of symptoms (du Toit et al., 2019). Screening and early diagnosis of dementia are essential to enable prisoners to receive the health and social care they are entitled to and in comparison with those living in the community. The importance of initial cognitive screening of prisoners in reception and at the beginning of their sentence by a healthcare professional commences this process, as well as building trust between the prisoner and healthcare professional when they first arrive in prison. However, the barriers and challenges of a cognitive screening of prisoners and diagnosing of dementia in a person with dementia are complex and have been discussed in more detail in Chapter 4.

Beyond the initial cognitive screening of prisoners, there is a need to continue cognitive screening during the course of the prison sentence, especially for sentences over five years for prisoners who are over the age of 50 (Combalbert et al., 2018). Currently, in the UK, continued cognitive screening has not been implemented. However, an important ethical consideration of cognitive screening, whether the person is within prison or living in the community, is that cognitive screening can only be completed when the individual has provided consent. This element has not been emphasised in published research illuminating the need for the development of an ethical framework. However, ethically, consent needs to be obtained from each individual before completing either cognitive screening or assessment.

Once a prisoner has been diagnosed with dementia, both pharmacological and non-pharmacological treatment options should be offered (Maschi et al., 2012). These treatments have been discussed in more detail in Chapter 3. However, for the requirements of the ethical guidelines provided for both prison healthcare settings and best practice in dementia care, consent from the prisoner should be obtained before treatment is provided. The involvement of prisoners with dementia in the development of treatment plans promotes their autonomy, which must be respected in the prison setting. Encouragement from healthcare professionals and prison staff working in prisons to support the prisoner with dementia to communicate their preferences for treatment decisions should be prioritised, ensuring an autonomous approach.

2 Ethical decisions and patient decision-making competence

A fundamental element of autonomy is for the individual to be empowered to make their own decisions. It is essential for healthcare professionals to complete a functional assessment to determine if a patient is capable of making a specific decision. In the UK, this is supported through the Mental Capacity Act 2005, as described in Chapter 2. It is important to recognise that it cannot be assumed that people with dementia do not have capacity to consent. All people with dementia will have the ability to indicate and make some decisions; the assessment of capacity needs to be situation-specific and relating to the particular decision under consideration (Hegde and Ellajosyula, 2016). The assessment must include four elements: communication, the patient can express their choice; understanding, the patient can recall information and link important elements; appreciation, the patient understands the outcomes of each possible decision; and rationalisation, the patient can weigh up the risks and benefits of the impact of the decision (Dastidar and Odden, 2011). The added complication for prisoners with dementia is a lack of training and education of prison and legal staff to support and enable prisoners to make informed situation-specific decisions, which needs to be addressed to support the balance of autonomy of prisoners with dementia and act in their best interests.

3 Information and disclosure

Information and disclosure of health information within a prison setting need careful consideration, especially as a diagnosis of dementia is associated with the assumption of loss of capacity, which will leave prisoners vulnerable. The disclosure of health information of prisoners to the prison administration is prohibited unless the prisoner provided explicit consent, as discussed more fully earlier in this chapter (Lehtmets and Pont, 2014). The only exception to this rule is a court order, when the healthcare professional communicates directly with a judge, or in rare cases when confidentiality needs to be breached due to the health and safety of the prisoner or others. However, to support prisoners with dementia, the sharing of information of a diagnosis to prison staff will enable staff to understand an individual prisoner and ensure their behaviour is not reprimanded, and the prisoner's health, safety and well-being is maintained during their prison sentence.

4 Recognising personhood

In the Nuffield Council on Bioethics' (2009) ethical framework, one component considers recognising personhood. This identifies that people living with dementia should be as equally valued as they were before their diagnosis, and this should continue throughout the course of their illness experience, regardless of cognitive and behavioural changes. Thus, the person with dementia is still the same person as before onset, and this should guide policy for people living with dementia in the community. The element of personhood and people with dementia receiving person-centred care is explored in depth in Chapter 3, and the difficulties of providing this approach within a prison setting and a strict regime becomes apparent. This should not affect the level of care received by prisoners with dementia; issues such as these are rarely to the benefit of politicians and are therefore often neglected in public policy and funding (du Toit et al., 2019). However, there are a number of prisons around the world who have begun to address and recognise the personhood of prisoners, including those with dementia, and have implemented various initiatives as explored within Chapter 4.

5 Family involvement

The role of families in dementia care within the community is recognised within all the existing guidelines regarding ethics of healthcare in dementia. There is currently a lack of information on how family members can be involved in supporting relatives with dementia in prison settings, and empirical research in this area is required. The role of family members is important when decisions need to be made with regard to the prisoner's treatment plan or accessing specialist care (Maschi et al., 2012; Treacy et al., 2019). However, this needs to be performed sensitively in a way that promotes the autonomy and interests of the prisoner with dementia, seeking consent for such involvement whilst also ensuring the prisoner with dementia is being provided with the care they are entitled to and that meets their needs. A suggestion to increase the liaison between the prisoner with dementia and their family and friends in order for the prisoner to feel supported has been offered, thus, enabling relationships that are meaningful to the prisoner with dementia, giving them the support they need in sustaining their sense of self and their values (Treacy et al., 2019).

A further ethical issue is the power of attorney and the need for family members of prisoners with dementia to obtain, where appropriate, power of attorney for both health and welfare and financial affairs. Decisions regarding power of attorney need to be made whilst the prisoner with dementia is able to understand the implications of supporting the family member to act in their best interests. These processes will support open communication between the prisoner with dementia, their family members and healthcare professionals. When there is no power of attorney in place, or no family members, there will be a dilemma of who should be the proxy for the prisoner with dementia. The added complexity of a prisoner with dementia could also result in the prison staff being responsible for making sure that the person living with dementia is having their best interests met and not circumvented by third parties. These considerations need to be addressed within an ethical framework for prisoners with dementia and their families to receive care that is humane and just.

6 Care and evaluation of care

Dementia is a progressive terminal illness, and therefore care provided to prisoners with dementia needs to be continually evaluated to ensure their changing needs are being met. Ethical challenges of long-term management of progressive diseases have been acknowledged when caring for patients in the community (Vaszar et al., 2002; MacKenzie and de Melo-Martin, 2015). One of the ethical challenges is the provision of care, including the evaluation of care and decisions on future care. Decisions regarding care for a person with a progressive illness may challenge their autonomy, especially in the case of dementia, as care includes not only health but personal and societal dimensions, and the involvement of a multidisciplinary team to support all of these elements (MacKenzie and de Melo-Martin, 2015). When the disease progresses, health and social care professionals, working with the patient and family will need to plan care that involves various combinations of initiating, withholding and withdrawing life-sustaining interventions, whilst adhering to the ethical principles of autonomy, beneficence, non-maleficence and justice (Vaszar et al., 2002).

These challenges are complicated when considering a person with dementia, and further complicated when that person is in prison. Because of the progressive nature of dementia, aspects of care need to be regularly assessed, developed and implemented to address the risks associated with its progression. An example is that of malnutrition, which may be caused due to difficulties with eating, such as poor motor coordination, lack of recognition of food or swallowing difficulties. The risk associated with the lack of recognition of swallowing is the development of pneumonia, which is accompanied by breathlessness and pain (Mitchell et al., 2009). The assessment and evaluation of care also needs to address the issue of when it is necessary to provide the patient with palliative and end-of-life care, and for prisoners, this needs to include the provision of hospice services (Imhof and Kaskie, 2008). Thus, for care that is ethical to be offered, skilled healthcare professionals are required within the prison setting to complete risk assessments and a care plan to fulfil their duty of care (Brooke et al., 2018).

7 Environment

The physical environment can become complex and daunting for people with dementia and have a negative impact on their independence and ability to maintain a good quality of life (Maschi et al., 2012; NHS, 2018). Prisoners with dementia also face a variety of potentially stressful environment features within the prison setting, such as overcrowding, lack of privacy, as well as architectural and structural challenges of the building, which often fail to support older prisoners, and especially those with dementia (Peacock et al., 2019). Environmental challenges for people with dementia exacerbate their levels of stress (Bedard et al., 2016). Within the prison environment, this stress could lead to agitation and disruption of the prison regime and potential reprimands for the prisoner. Therefore, the ethical perspective of ensuring no harm to oneself or harm to others needs to be considered, and healthcare professionals need to understand and assess the risks of harm to and by prisoners with dementia.

An important element is the adaptation of current prison environments to support and accommodate people with dementia, modifying both social and physical environments (Dillon et al., 2019; Patterson et al., 2014). This approach would also support older prisoners without dementia, and prisoners with disabilities, and is preferred to the transferring prisoners with dementia to specialised units, which would cause them further confusion (Patterson et al., 2014). Adaptations to prison environments need to be based on the dementia-friendly environment principles, which improve the utility of space for people with dementia (Department of Health, 2012; Department of Health, 2015; Peacock et al., 2019). Dementia-friendly environment principles promote understanding, respect and support to those who have dementia (Department of Health, 2012). In the prison setting, these might include design features that promote safety as well as encouraging social interaction and activities (Peacock et al., 2019). However, a prison setting is still a challenging environment for someone who is severely ill and the ethical questions surrounding the continuation of the sentence must be raised (du Toit et al., 2019; Maschi et al., 2012).

Another approach to support older prisoners, who cannot manage in the mainstream environment of prison because of old buildings, uneven floors and cast-iron stairs, is the development of specialised units. These units house older prisoners and those with physical disabilities, who may or may not have dementia, and are a way of supporting this population separate from mainstream prison environment and population (Atabay, 2009). However, consideration needs to given as to the management of the behaviours that may manifest as a result of dementia. Specialised units would need to demonstrate the ability to cope with displays of aggression and/or confusion without imposing penalties (Moll, 2013). In addition, as explored in Chapter 2, dementia is not a normal part of aging, and therefore grouping older prisoners together and those with dementia may be disruptive rather than beneficial. Transferring prisoners to specialist units may also involve moving the prisoners further away from their families and this could increase their confusion and agitation (du Toit et al., 2019). Further discussion and research are required around the benefits of specialist units to ensure this approach is applicable, supportive and beneficial to prisoners with dementia.

8 Training for prison staff

The ethical issues of dementia care discussed in the second part of this chapter illuminate the diverse and complex experiences of the main triad involved in dementia care: the person with dementia, their family members supporting them and health and social care professionals. The work of Strech et al. (2013) provides an evidence-based overview of the breadth of ethical issues and need for all of these to be recognised in clinical practice, to support the person with dementia, their family members and health and social care professionals. These ethical issues also need to be recognised in prison settings and understood by all those who work and live in this environment. Therefore, an understanding of dementia and how to support a prisoner with dementia expands beyond that of health and social care professionals and includes prison staff, officers and even other prisoners.

Ethically, it is important to recognise and support rather than reprimand a prisoner's behaviours that are beyond their control due to dementia. However, prison staff report a lack of training to develop their skills to identify and support prisoners with dementia (Dillon et al., 2019). Studies exploring the knowledge of dementia by those who work with prisoners have only just commenced. However, the overwhelming recommendation from this new body of work is the need for further education and training for all staff and prisoners who come into contact with prisoners with dementia (Brooke et al., 2018; Dillon et al., 2019; du Toit et al., 2019; Peacock et al., 2019), in particular, education and training regarding how to identify symptoms of dementia that supports the case for a medical referral, how to support dementia-associated behaviours and how to detect changes in symptoms as the disease progresses (Maschi et al., 2012).

A robust prison-specific dementia education workshop has been developed, through a three-phase research-based study (Brooke and Rybacka, 2020). Phases 1 and 2 involved understanding staff's and prisoners' knowledge of dementia, barriers and current initiatives to support prisoners with dementia. Phase 3 involved the development and implementation of a two-hour dementia education workshop from the knowledge and experiences of staff and prisoners. The prison-specific dementia education workshop has been delivered to staff, prisoners and volunteers and has been received well, and all who attended fully engaged in the process with informed discussions, which challenged many misconceptions (Brooke and Rybacka, 2020). However, this has only been developed and delivered in the Prison Service of England and Wales.

Summary

This chapter introduced the four principles of medical ethics, beneficence, non-maleficence, autonomy and justice; the UN Principles of Medical Ethics; and the challenges of the applications of an ethical approach to healthcare in prison settings, including confidentiality, consent and a duty of care. The delivery of healthcare in a prison setting is clearly influenced by the prison environment, which hinders and creates a significant challenge to the provision of equitable healthcare, as compared to wider society. Ethical healthcare for people with dementia has been introduced, and the need to do the morally right thing with many options and none unambiguously right has been discussed. Complex ethical issues within dementia care have been acknowledged, and a framework has been developed to support an ethical approach to dementia care. Finally, the care for people with dementia in prison was explored with the development of an ethical framework, which illuminates ethical practices of merging guidelines into practice and offers a starting point for future research.

References

Alperovitch, A., Dreifuss-Netter, F., Dickele, A.M., Gaudray, P., Le Cox, P., Rouvillois, P., et al. (2009). *Ethical Issues Raised by a Possible Influenza Pandemic, National Consultative Ethics Committee for Health and Life Sciences*. April 3. Available from: www.ccne-ethique.fr/sites/default/files/publications/avis_106_anglais.pdf [Accessed on: 22 May 2020].

Alzheimer Europe (2010). *The Four Common Bioethical Principles*. Available from: www.alzheimer-europe.org/Ethics/Definitions-and-approaches/The-four-common-bioethical-principles/Justice [Accessed on: 22 May 2020].

Atabay, T. (2009). Older prisoners. In *Handbook on Prisoners with Special Needs. Criminal Justice Handbook Series* (pp. 123–143). Vienna, Austria: United Nations.

Bavidge, M. (2006). Aging and human nature. In J.C. Hughes (Ed.) *Dementia: Mind, Meaning, and the Person* (pp. 41–53). Oxford: Oxford University Press.

Beauchamp, T.L. (1989). *Medical Ethics: The Moral Responsibilities of Physicians* (p. 195). Englewood Cliffs, NJ: Prentice-Hall.

Beauchamp, T.L., Childress, J.F. (2001). *Principles of Biomedical Ethics*. 5th edition. Oxford: Oxford University Press.

Bedard, R., Metzger, L., Williams, B. (2016). Ageing prisoners: an introduction to geriatric health-care challenges in correctional facilities. *International Review of the Red Cross*, 98(903): 917–939.

Brooke, J.M., Diaz-Gil, A., Jackson, D. (2018). The impact of dementia in the prison setting: a systematic review. *Dementia*, 19(5): 1509–1531.

Brooke, J.M., Kirk, M. (2014). Advance care planning in patients with dementia. *British Journal of Community Nursing*, 19(10): 422–427.

Brooke, J.M., Rybacka, M. (2020). Development of a dementia education workshop for prison staff, prisoners, and health and social care professionals to enable them to support prisoners with dementia. *Journal of Correctional Health Care*, DOI: 10.1177/1078345820916444.

Combalbert, N., Pennequin, V., Ferrance, C., Armand, M., Anselme, M., Geffray, B. (2018). Cognitive impairment, self-perceived health and quality of life of older prisoners. *Criminal Behaviour and Mental Health*, 28(1): 36–49.

Council of Europe (1993). *Health Care Services in Prisons. European Committee for the Prevention of Torture and Inhuman or Degrading Treatment or Punishment (CPT)*. Available from: https://rm.coe.int/16806ce943 [Accessed on: 22 May 2020].

Council of Europe (2006). *European Prison Rules*. Available from: https://rm.coe.int/european-prison-rules-978-92-871-5982-3/16806ab9ae [Accessed on: 22 May 2020].

Council of Europe (2020). *About the CPT. Health Care Services in Prisons. European Committee for the Prevention of Torture and Inhuman or Degrading Treatment or Punishment (CPT)*. Available from: www.coe.int/en/web/cpt/faqs [Accessed on: 22 May 2020].

Dastidar, J.G., Odden, A. (2011). How do I determine if my patient has decision-making capacity? *The Hospitalist*, 8.

Department of Health (2012). *Prime Minister's Challenge on Dementia: Delivering Major Improvements in Dementia Care and Research by 2015*. London: Department of Health.

Department of Health (2015). *Prime Minister's Challenge on Dementia 2020*. London: Department of Health.

Dillon, G., Vinter, L.P., Winder, B., Finch, L. (2019). 'The guy might not even be able to remember why he's here and what he's in here for and why he's locked in': residents and prison staff experiences of living and working alongside people with dementia who are serving prison sentences for a sexual offence. *Psychology, Crime and Law*, 25(5): 440–457.

du Toit, S.H.J., Withall, A., O'Loughlin, K., Ninaus, N., Lovarini, M., Snoyman, P., Butler, T., Forsyth, K., Surr, C.A. (2019). Best care options for older prisoners with dementia: a scoping review. *International Psychogeriatrics*, 31(8): 1081–1097.

Ethical Practice (2020). *Registered Nursing*. Available from: www.registerednursing.org/nclex/ethical-practice/ [Accessed on: 22 May 2020].

Fazel, S., McMillan, J., O'Donnell, I. (2002). Dementia in prison: ethical and legal implications. *Journal of Medical Ethics*, 28: 156–159.

Galvin, K., Todres, L. (2011). Kinds of well-being: a conceptual framework that provides direction for caring. *International Journal of Qualitative Studies on Health and Well-Being*, 6(4): 10362.

Gatherer, A., Enggist, S., Møller, L. (2014). The essentials about prisons and health. In S. Enggist, L. Møller, G. Galea, C. Udeson (Eds.) *Prisons and Health*. Copenhagen: WHO Regional Office for Europe.

Gillon, R. (1994). Medical ethics: four principles plus attention to scope. *BMJ*, 309: 184–188.

Hegde, S., Ellajosyula, R. (2016). Capacity issues and decision-making in dementia. *Annals of Indian Academy of Neurology*, 19 (Supp11): S34–S39.

House of Commons, Health and Social Care Committee (2018). *Prison Health. Twelfth Report of Session 2017–19. Report, Together with Formal Minutes Relating to the Report*. Available from: https://publications.parliament.uk/pa/cm201719/cmselect/cmhealth/963/963.pdf [Accessed on: 22 May 2020].

Houtepen, R., ter Meulen, R.H.J. (2000). The expectations of solidarity: matters of justice, responsibility and identity in the reconstruction of the health care system. *Health Care Analysis*, 8: 355–376.

Hughes, J.C. (2002). Dementia and ethics: the view of informal carers. *Journal of the Royal Society of Medicine*, 95: 242–246.

Hughes, J.C., Hope, T., Reader, S., Rice, D. (2002). Dementia and ethics: the views of informal carers. *Journal of the Royal Society of Medicine*, 95: 242–246.

Hughes, J.C., Sabat, S.R. (2008). The advance directive conjuring trick and the person with dementia. In G. Widdershoven, J. McMillan, T. Hope (Eds.) *Empirical Ethics in Psychiatry* (pp. 123–140). Oxford: Oxford University Press.

Imhof, S., Kaskie, B. (2008). How can we make the pain go away? Public policies to manage pain at the end of life. *Gerontologist*, 48: 423–431.

International Covenant on Civil and Political Rights (1976). *United Nations Human Rights Office of the High Commissioner*, 2 May 2020. Available from: www.ohchr.org/EN/Professionallnterest/Pages/CCPR.aspx [Accessed on: 22 May 2020].

International Covenant on Economic, Social and Cultural Rights (1976). *United Nations Human Rights Office of the High Commissioner.* Available from: www.ohchr.org/EN/profes sionalinterest/pages/cescr.aspx [Accessed on: 22 May 2020].

Kinsinger, F.S. (2010). Beneficence and the professional's moral imperative. *Journal of Chiro-practic Humanities,* 16(1): 44–46.

Lehtmets, A., Pont, J. (2014). *A Manual for Health-Care Workers and Other Prison Staff with Responsibility for Prisoners' Well-Being.* Council of Europe. Available from: https://rm.coe. int/prisons-healthcare-and-medical-ethics-eng-2014/16806ab9b5 [Accessed on: 22 May 2020].

MacKenzie, C.R., de Melo-Martin, I. (2015). Ethical considerations in chronic musculo-skeletal disease. *Current Reviews in Musculoskeletal Medicine,* 8(2): 128–133.

Maschi, T., Kwak, J., Ko, E., Morrissey, M.B. (2012). Forget me not: dementia in prison. *The Gerontologist,* 52(4): 441–451.

Mental Welfare Commission for Scotland (2007). *Safe to Wander?* Edinburgh: Mental Wel-fare Commission for Scotland.

Miskelly, F. (2005). Electronic tracking of patients with dementia and wandering using mobile phone technology. *Age and Ageing,* 34: 497–518.

Mitchell, S.L., Teno, J.M., Kiely, D.K., Shaffer, M.L., Jones, R.N., Prigerson, H.G., Volicer, L. (2009). The clinical course of advanced dementia. *The New England Journal of Medicine,* 361(16): 1529–1538.

Moll, A. (2013). *Losing Track of Time. Dementia and the Ageing Prison Population: Treatment Challenges and Examples of Good Practice.* London: Mental Health Foundation.

Munyaradzi, M. (2012). Critical reflections on the principle of beneficence in biomedicine. *The Pan African Medical Journal.* Available from: www.panafrican-med-journal.com/con tent/article/11/29/full/ [Accessed on: 22 May 2020].

National Health Service (2018). *How to Make Your Home Dementia Friendly. Dementia Guide,* June 4, 2020. Available from: www.nhs.uk/conditions/dementia/home-environment/ [Accessed on: 22 May 2020].

Niemeijer, A.R., Frederiks, B.J.M., Riphagen, I.I., Legemaate, J., Eefsting, J.A., Hertogh, C.M.P.M. (2010). Ethical and practical concerns of surveillance technologies in residen-tial care for people with dementia or intellectual disabilities: an overview of the literature. *International Psychogeriatric,* 22(7): 1129–1142.

Nuffield Council on Bioethics (2009). *Dementia: Ethical Issues.* London: Cambridge Publishers.

Oliver, D., Gee, P. (2009). Communication, barriers to it and information sharing. In G. Rai (Ed.) *Medical Ethics and the Elderly* (pp. 49–61). Oxford: Radcliffe.

Patterson, K., Newman, C., Doona, K. (2014). Improving the care of older persons in Aus-tralian prisons using the Policy Delphi method. *Dementia,* 15(5): 1219–1233.

Peacock, S.C., Burles, M., Hodson, A., Kumaran, M., MacRae, R., Peternelj-Taylor, C., Holtslander, L. (2019). Older person with dementia in prison: an integrative review. *Inter-national Journal of Prisoner Health,* 16(1): 1–16.

Penal Reform International (2001). *Making Standards Work. An International Handbook on Good Prison Practice.* 2nd edition. Available from: www.penalreform.org [Accessed on: 22 May 2020].

Pont, J. (2006). Medical ethics in prisons: rules, standards and challenges. *International Journal of Prisoner Health,* 2(4): 259–267.

Pont, J. (2011). *Medical Ethics in Prison.* Conference Presentation. Available from: www. unodc.org/documents/balticstates/EventsPresentations/FinalConf_24-25Mar11/ Pont_25_March.pdf [Accessed on: 22 May 2020].

Pont, J., Stöver, H., Gétaz, L., Casillas, A., Wolff, H. (2015). Prevention of violence in prison – *The Role of Health Care Professionals. Journal of Forensic and Legal Medicine*, 34: 127–132.

Pont, J., Stöver, H., Wolff, H. (2012). Resolving ethical conflicts in practice and research. *Health Policy and Ethics*, e1–e6.

Pratt, C., Schmall, V., Wright, S. (1987). Ethical concerns of family caregivers to dementia patients. *The Gerontological Society of America*, 27(5): 632–638.

Prison and Probation Ombudsman (2017). *Annual Report 2016–2017*. Available from: https://s3-eu-west-2.amazonaws.com/ppo-prod-storage-1g9rkhjhkjmgw/uploads/2017/07/PPO_Annual-Report-201617_Interactive.pdf [Accessed on: 22 May 2020].

Rabins, P.V. (2007). Can suicide be a rational and ethical act in persons with early or pre-dementia? *American Journal of Bioethics*, 7: 47–49.

Rabins, P.V., Black, B.S. (2010). Ethical issues in geriatric psychiatry. *International Review of Psychiatry*, 22: 267–273.

Sacristán, J.A., Aguaron, A., Avendaño-Solá, C., et al. (2016). Patient involvement in clinical research: why, when and how. *Patient Preference and Adherence*, 10: 631–640.

Strech, D., Mertz, M., Knüppel, H., Neitzke, G., Schmidhuber, M. (2013). The full spectrum of ethical issues in dementia care: systematic qualitative review. *The British Journal of Psychiatry*, 202: 400–406.

Todres, L., Galvin, K. (2006). Caring for a partner with Alzheimer's disease: intimacy, loss and the life that is possible. *International Journal of Qualitative Studies on Health and Well-Being*, 1(1): 50–61.

Treacy, S., Haggith, A., Wickramasinghe, N.D., Van Bortel, T. (2019). Dementia-friendly prisons: a mixed-methods evaluation of the application of dementia-friendly community principles to two prisons in England. *BMJ Open*, 9: e030087.

United Nations (1982). *Principles of Medical Ethics*. Available from: https://digitallibrary.un.org/record/43638?ln=en [Accessed on: 22 May 2020].

Vaszar, L.T., Weinacker, A.B., Henig, N.R., Raffin, T.A. (2002). Ethical issues in the long-term management of progressive degenerative neuromuscular diseases. *Seminars in Respiratory and Critical Care Medicine*, 23(3): 307–314.

World Health Organization (WHO) (2003). *Prison Health as Part of Public Health*. Declaration of Moscow, 24 October. Regional Office for Europe. Available from: www.euro.who.int/Document/HIPP/newsletter-apr04-eng.pdf [Accessed on: 22 May 2020].

World Medical Association (1948). *Declaration of Geneva*. Geneva, Switzerland.

7 Research in prison

Joanne Brooke and Monika Rybacka

Historical context of research in prison

There is a need for an overview of the historical context of research in the prison environment, as during the last century research with prisoners repeatedly ignored ethical considerations, which led to the exploitation of prisoners and research that resulted in their mistreatment and death. The focus of this section is on research that mainly occurred in the USA and Germany, but it is acknowledged that research on prisoners occurred within the timeframe discussed around the world.

Reports documenting biomedical experimentation in prisons, which severely violated human rights date back as early as 1906 and 1912, when Dr Strong in Bilibid Prison in Manila caused the death of prisoners through his experiments exploring cholera and beriberi, although prisoners who survived were provided with cigars and cigarettes (Hornblum, 1998). In 1915, prisoners in Mississippi State Penitentiary were asked to participate in an experiment exploring the causes of pellagra. This research occurred even though doctors had known since 1735 the cause of pellagra was malnutrition, which raised question of why the study was conducted at all. However, 11 prisoners were starved until they showed signs of malnutrition, with the promise of being released from prison if they agreed to participate (Goldberger and Wheeler, 1915). During the early nineteenth century, prisoners who volunteered to be subjects in medical research were often granted freedom if they survived, including those serving life sentences. Between 1919 and 1922, Dr Stanley performed testicular transplant experiments on 500 prisoners at San Quentin State Prison in California, inserting the testicles of recently executed prisoners and goats into the scrotums of living prisoners or 'mashing' the testicles to inject the mixture into the prisoner's abdomen. Dr Stanley believed that disease caused crime, and that murderers probably had overdeveloped thyroids and those who committed forgery had underdeveloped pituitary glands (Lederer, 1995; Stanley, 1922).

Isolated incidents of prison-based research before World War II formed the foundation for a practice that would become firmly embedded in the structure of American clinical research during World War II. Perhaps the most significant wartime medical research project in which American scientists recruited prisoners as research subjects occurred in Illinois's Statesville Prison. In the beginning of 1942, hundreds of Illinois prisoners were exposed to cases of malaria, as researchers attempted to find more effective means to prevent and cure tropical diseases that ravaged Allied forces in the Pacific (Alving et al., 1948). Prisoners were informed they were helping the war effort and not that they were going to be intentionally infected with a potentially fatal disease. Later in 1942, researchers injected 64 Massachusetts prisoners with cow's blood in a Navy-sponsored experiment; the rejection of this foreign material by the prisoners was catastrophic (Fitzpatrick, 2012). In 1944, a well-known microbiologist, performed experiments on four volunteer prisoners from the state prison at Dearborn, Michigan, inoculating them with hepatitis-infected specimens obtained in North Africa (Newman, 2005). One prisoner died; two others developed hepatitis but survived and the fourth developed severe symptoms but did not actually contract the disease. In a follow-up study in the 1950s, 200 female prisoners were infected with viral hepatitis to study the disease (Hornblum, 1998).

The exploitation and abuse of prisoners culminated during the World War II, including the Nazi concentration camps and the Japanese Unit 731. The prisoners were subjected to experiments on high altitude, freezing, sea water, malaria, epidemic jaundice, spotted fever, typhoid, bubonic plague, anthrax, tissue regeneration and transplantation, mustard gas, incendiary bombs and biological weapons, resulting in an excessive number of deaths (Annas and Grodin, 1992). There are also reports on research involving US prisoners during World War II on malaria, sand fly fever, dengue fever, sleeping sickness, gonorrhoea, gas gangrene and beef blood injections (Hornblum, 1998). Some, but not all, of these experiments were aimed at gaining knowledge for military purposes. The crimes of the Nazi doctors were the subject of the Doctors' Trial during the Nuremberg Trial and gave rise to the Nuremberg Code on research involving humans (Annas and Grodin, 1992).

The Nuremberg Code is the most important document in the history of the ethics of medical research (Annas and Grodin, 1992). The code was formulated in 1947 in Nuremberg, Germany, by American, British, French and USSR judges sitting in judgement of Nazi doctors in what was called the Doctors' Trial. The Nazi doctors were accused of conducting human experiments in the concentration camps that involved torture and led to death. The Nuremberg Code provided the basic principles that stated the rights of subjects in medical research (Moreno, 1997). It contains ten principles, which focus on the explicit and voluntary consent of subjects involved in experiments. The principles include informed consent, absence of coercion and beneficence towards participants (Weindling, 2001).

Nuremberg Code (1947)

1   The voluntary consent of the human subject is absolutely essential.
2   The experiment should be such as to yield fruitful results for the good of society, unprocurable by other methods or means of study, and not random and unnecessary in nature.

3 The experiment should be so designed and based on the results of animal experimentation and a knowledge of the natural history of the disease or other problem under study that the anticipated results will justify the performance of the experiment.

4 The experiment should be so conducted as to avoid all unnecessary physical and mental suffering and injury.

5 No experiment should be conducted where there is *a priori* reason to believe that death or disabling injury will occur; except, perhaps, in those experiments where the experimental physicians also serve as subjects.

6 The degree of risk to be taken should never exceed that determined by the humanitarian importance of the problem to be solved by the experiment.

7 Proper preparations should be made and adequate facilities provided to protect the experimental subject against even remote possibilities of injury, disability, or death.

8 The experiment should be conducted only by scientifically qualified persons. The highest degree of skill and care should be required through all stages of the experiment of those who conduct or engage in the experiment

9 During the course of the experiment the human subject should be at liberty to bring the experiment to an end if he has reached the physical or mental state where continuation of the experiment seems to him to be impossible.

10 During the course of the experiment the scientist in charge must be prepared to terminate the experiment at any stage, if he has probable cause to believe, in the exercise of the good faith, superior skill and careful judgment required of him that a continuation of the experiment is likely to result in injury, disability, or death to the experimental subject.

Despite the Nuremberg Code being developed by US experts who were present at Nuremberg, it was US prisoners who after World War II became victims of further scientific exploitation by the rapidly evolving biomedical research and pharmaceutical industry. Prisoners again were infected with contagious material (histoplasmosis, infectious hepatitis, syphilis, amoebic dysentery, malaria, influenza), injected with living cancer cells and subjected to radiation and toxic agents (Hornblum, 1998). In 1952, Dr Southam injected live cancer calls into prisoners at the Ohio State Prison to study the progression of the disease (Langer, 1964). In 1956, Dr Sabin tested an experimental polio vaccine on 133 prisoners in Ohio (Hornblum, 1998).

During the 1960s, prisoners in the Colorado State Penitentiary were used as subjects in an experiment designed to determine the survival time and characteristics of red blood cells during periods of rapid red cell formation and during periods of severe iron deficiency. This process was achieved by red cells transfused into recipients, which were tagged with either radioactive iron or radioactive phosphorus (ACHRE Report, 1996). Between 1965 and 1966, Dr Kligman exposed approximately 75 prisoners at Holmesburg prison to high doses of dioxin, the main poisonous ingredient in Agent Orange (Hornblum,

1998). A chemical company had paid Dr Kligman to conduct the experiments to explore the toxicity effects of this chemical warfare agent. Dr Kligman exposed prisoners to a dosage 468 times greater than what was in the protocol for the experiments (Reiter, 2009). Other government-sponsored experiments on prisoners were conducted, such as in Oklahoma State Penitentiary where routine metabolic studies of experimental drugs using tracer amounts of radionuclides occurred, in Statesville Prison in Illinois where measurements of radium burden received from drinking water was investigated, and in San Quentin prison in California where researchers tracked the movement of iron from plasma to red blood cells using a radioactive marker (Appleman, 2020).

Two significant radiation experiments were held in Oregon and Washington prisons. In 1963, Carl Heller was a medical scientist in the field of endocrinology and was provided funding to review the effects of radiation on male reproductive function (Heller, 1963). Heller designed a study to test the effects of radiation on the somatic and germinal cells of the testes, including the dose required to produce change or induce damage to the spermatogenic cells, the length of time for cell production to recover and the effects of radiation on hormone excretion (Hornblum, 1998).

In 1963 in Oregon, using prisoners as research subjects was an accepted practice. In this Carl Heller's study, Oregon law was interpreted by state officials as permitting an inmate to give his consent to a vasectomy and was analogous to consenting to becoming an experimental research subject (ACHRE Report, 1996). However, important ethical concerns such as balancing risks and benefits, the quality of informed consent and subject-selection criteria were not addressed by the investigators or those responsible. Evidence suggests the quality of consent was poor, as many if not most of the subjects were not aware of the small risk of testicular cancer, the significant pain associated with the biopsies and the possible long-term effects. Regarding potential health benefits to the subjects, there were none, and the prisoners who volunteered for the research were apparently informed of this. However, the prisoners were offered financial incentives, which could be considered as coercion.

In January 1973, in a rapidly changing research ethics environment, the Oregon radiation experiments were terminated by the US Corrections Division, as it was concluded that prisoners could not consent freely to participate as subjects (Boly, 1977). In 1976, a number of subjects filed lawsuits effectively alleging poorly supervised research and lack of informed consent. In their depositions, they alleged that fellow prisoners had sometimes controlled the radiation dose to which they were exposed, that a prisoner with a grudge against a subject filled a syringe with water instead of Novocain, resulting in a vasectomy performed without anaesthetic and that the experimental procedures resulted in considerable pain and discomfort for which they were not prepared (Marini et al., 1976).

In a Washington prison, Dr Paulsen followed in the footsteps of Dr Heller and directed a substantial research program of his own. Dr Paulsen received a grant from the Atomic Energy Commission to study the effects of ionising radiation on testicular function (ACHRE Report, 1996). A significant differ- ence between the projects was that Dr Paulsen planned to move from X-rays to neutron irradiation (Chancellor et al., 2018). However, this part of the research was never completed. Dr Paulsen's project was terminated in 1970 because of concerns about the greater risks of exposing participants to neutron irradiation. Dr Paulsen did not inform the prisoners that they were required to undergo a vasectomy at the end of the experiment to ensure that subjects did not father 'genetically damaged children' (ACHRE Report, 1996). Both doctors viewed prisoners as ideal subjects – healthy, adult males who were not going anywhere (ACHRE Report, 1996).

In 1963, few researchers had any concerns about using prisoners as research subjects. However, Dr Maurice Pappworth demanded ethical behaviour in hos- pitals and cited examples of medical misconduct in his book 'Human Guinea Pig' (1967). Dr Pappworth was considered to be a whistleblower, shedding light on unethical experiments that were being conducted without the full knowledge of the prisoner. The Human Guinea Pig detailed experiments on children, prisoners in mental and penal institutions, as well as other vulnerable patients whose lives were often damaged. Dr Pappworth argued these vulner- able subjects were used to enhance the careers of the medics involved and dedi- cated an entire chapter of his book to the vulnerability of prisoners. There was an increasing gradual change in public opinion regarding the vulnerability of prisoners, which prompted new legislation to restrict prison research. By 1973, ethicists, researchers and others stated that incarcerated people were recognised as a vulnerable population and in an environment where they were unlikely to be able to give voluntary consent (Smoyer et al., 2009).

In 1976, the United States National Commission for the Protection of Human Subjects of Biomedical and Behavioural Research, created as a result of the National Research Act of 1974, with support from the Department of Health, Education and Welfare (DHEW) produced the DHEW Report (1976). This report gave an overview of the nature and extent of research involving prisoners. It was developed through prison visits and public hearings and discussed findings from philosophical, sociological, behavioural and legal perspectives. The commission raised two significant concerns about the use of prisoners as research subjects. The first was whether prisoners bear a fair share of the burdens and receive a fair share of the benefits of research. The second was whether prisoners are, in the words of the Nuremberg Code, 'so situated as to be able to exercise free power of choice', and if they were in a position to provide voluntary consent to participate in research. These two concerns related to two ethical principles: the principle of justice, which requires that persons and groups be treated fairly; and the principle of autonomy, which emphasises the need to promote and respect an individual's decision. The com- mission stated that the disproportionate use of prisoners in certain kinds of research (e.g. phase 1 drug testing) would constitute a violation of the first principle and the closed and coercive prison environment would compromise the second principle.

The commission made several recommendations that focused on the minimal or no risk to the prisoners involved in the research, the intent of the research having reasonable probability of improving the health or well-being of the participating prisoners and that the research will be reviewed by a national ethical review body for suitability of the research and the researchers themselves. The DHEW Report (1976) and its recommendations influenced the American federal government to apply regulations to research involving prisoners and to limit prison research to narrow categories of non-intrusive, low-risk, individually beneficial research (Hornblum, 1998; Reiter, 2009).

The DHEW Report (1976) was followed by the Belmont Report (Office for Human Research Protection, 1979). The Belmont Report was written by the National Commission for the Protection of Human Subjects of Biomedical and Behavioural Research. The commission was charged with identifying the basic ethical principles that should underlie the conduct of biomedical and behavioural research involving any human subjects (not just prisoners) and developing specific guidelines to ensure that such research is conducted in accordance with those principles, building on the recommendations set out in the DHEW Report (1976). The report was informed by monthly discussions that spanned four years and an intensive four days of deliberation in 1976. The commission published the Belmont Report in 1979, which identifies basic ethical principles and guidelines that address ethical issues arising from the conduct of research with human subjects.

By 1978, two of the largest pharmaceutical companies had ceased phase 1 drug trials in Michigan state prisons, and simultaneously state prisons stopped doctors like Dr. Kligman from completing research programs in their prisons (Reiter, 2009). However, 40 years after Dr. Kligman conducted dioxin experiments and 30 years after the DHEW Report (1976) and Belmont Report (1979), prisoners continued to be used in medical experiments. Most recently between 2006 and 2008, a drug company contracted with jurisdictions in several USA states to enrol criminal defendants in an experimental drug addiction treatment programme. State judges sentenced criminal defendants who had been found in possession of drugs into an experimental treatment programme that involved 30 days of treatment with three different drugs, none of which had been approved for addiction treatment by the Food and Drug Administration (Reiter, 2009). In 2006, the Department of Health and Human Services commissioned the Institute of Medicine to re-evaluate the federal standards governing medical experimentation on prisoners (Gostin et al., 2007). The Institute of Medicine (Gostin et al., 2007) reported a need for significant changes in the ethical standards governing medical experiments on prisoners. The report recommends streamlining and expanding oversight of prisoner experimentation and replacing the current categorical limitations on prisoner experimentation with case-by-case risk-benefit analyses of individual experiments.

Protecting prisoners from exploitation

The history of health research on prisoners, without their consent or even their knowledge, as described previously, has subsequently led to prisoners becoming overprotected and understudied (Moser et al., 2004; Cislo and Trestman, 2013). Legislation has been implemented in the majority of countries around the world to prevent exploitation of prisoners through research, which includes the restriction of research funding (Christopher et al., 2011). Only studies which pose no more than a minimal risk to prisoners who participate have been allowed to proceed. This was because of the belief that prisoners would be unable to provide informed consent due to their lack of autonomy from the removal of their liberty (Gostin et al., 2007). Therefore, in the late 1990s, prisoners were only included in 15 per cent of all clinical health research in the US (Hoffman, 2000).

Currently, there still remains a lack of health research in the prison setting (Ahalt et al., 2012, 2015), and research that does occur does not necessarily recruit prisoners but entails a review of custodial health records. This approach prevents an in-depth understanding of prisoners' health needs (Ahalt et al., 2017) and the development of evidence-based interventions to support and improve prisoners' health (Kouyoumdjian et al., 2015; Kouyoumdjian et al., 2015b). Although this is beginning to change, there is a need for research to develop evidence-based healthcare in prison settings. Evidence-based healthcare will inform a healthcare professional's clinical decision making to support prisoners' physical and mental health whilst in prison, which is essential. However, the protection of prisoners from exploitation with regard to participating in research is not a straightforward task (Christopher et al., 2016). The following sections will include the discussion of a transactional framework of exploitation (Wertheimer, 1999) and how this approach can be applied to understand when research with prisoners is exploitative. A number of important aspects will then be introduced, such as obtaining informed consent, the coercive prison environment and the ability of ensuring confidentiality.

When is research with prisoners exploitative?

The transactional framework of exploitation (Wertheimer, 1999) was applied to the exploitation of prisoners to participate in research by Christopher et al. (2016). The transactional framework states exploitation occurs when one party (A) takes unfair advantage of another party (B), and this occurs when one of two conditions are met:

Condition one is the process of threatening harm; for example A can threaten B with a negative action or outcome, if B does not engage with A as requested. The application of this condition in research in a prison setting could be the threat of segregation or withdrawal of privileges; therefore A will be exploiting B.

Condition two occurs when A takes an unfair advantage of B, as the benefit for A is significant compared to the benefit for B. Unlike condition one, this condition does not always need to be prevented, as doing so may prevent B from attending some gain from the transaction that would otherwise not be possible. This form of exploitation may be acceptable if informed consent has been obtained from B, who will not be harmed, and B receives the expected benefit (Emanuel, 2008). The argument to accept condition two is that the comparison of the type and amount of benefit A and B receive is irrelevant; the importance is B views the benefit as acceptable. Exploitation under condition two can occur in research where A benefits more than B, for example B's (participant) involvement in a clinical trial for an experimental drug for A (a pharmaceutical company), as the participant may receive preferential treatment in the prison, and more intensive medical care, whilst the drug may not be available to prisoners on completion of the trial. Therefore, it could be argued that the pharmaceutical company benefits exceed those of the participant, but applying the transactional model of exploitation, this exploitation may be permissible if all other ethical conditions are met. However, this does not address the issue of coercion, which will be discussed later.

Currently, one contemporary study has explored a prisoner's decision-making process to participate in one of six different clinical trials (Christopher et al., 2016). A questionnaire to explore prisoners' views and beliefs of being exploited was developed, which included three types of exploitation; general, treatment, and a desire for access. The closed questionnaire included a seven-point Likert scale ranging from 1 – totally disagree to 7 – totally agree for eight questions, which included:

> General Exploitation: The study took advantage of the fact I was in prison; The researchers in this study used me to get what they wanted; I felt taken advantage of by being in this study; This study exploited me.
>
> Treatment Exploitation: Joining the study was the only way to get the treatment I needed; I only joined the study because I couldn't get the treatment I needed in prison.
>
> Desire for Access: There should be more research studies for prisoners to join if they want to; Inmates should have the chance to join more research studies.

Christopher et al. (2016) identified that the majority of prisoners did not feel exploited by participating in a clinical research trial, although prisoners were motivated by the access to healthcare, which they usually struggled to obtain. However, the interpretation of the questions needs to be considered, as Christopher et al. (2016) identified the first two general exploitation questions could be read as being factually true, without the prisoner feeling they were exploited by participating in the research. Applying the transactional framework of exploitation to the results of this questionnaire would suggest these studies did not involve unacceptable exploitation. However, even if prisoners thought the research was potentially exploitative, it was permissible and in some cases identified as desirable. A noted limitation of this study is that all the clinical research trials the prisoners had participated in adhered to the appropriate guidelines and posed minimal risk to the prisoners.

Practicalities of research in the prison setting

In Europe, the Additional Protocol to the Convention on Human Rights and Biomedicine, concerning Biomedical Research (Council of Europe, 2005) states that prisoners should be included in both beneficial and non-beneficial research, if non-beneficial research is particular to prisoners and the prison setting and offers group benefit with minimal risk. Prisoners should receive the same opportunity to participate in health research as other members of the population of the country they are detained (Charles and Draper, 2012). Therefore, the practicalities of research in the prison setting need to be addressed. Within this section, three important elements of research in a prison setting will be discussed, namely obtaining informed consent, the coercive prison environment and confidentiality. Each of these elements contains particular challenges unique to a prison setting, each of which are complex and require an in-depth understanding of these multi-dimensional challenges.

Consent

Informed consent is an essential and core element in research involving human beings. This is to ensure anyone participating in research is fully aware of the risks and benefits and volunteers free from any coercion. The acknowledgement of the need for informed consent in prison research was first raised in a report to the Governor of Illinois Stateville Penitentiary in 1948 (Ivy, 1948). The report identified three necessary components of consent: first, all participants should be able to freely volunteer without any coercion; second, all participants should understand the risks of the research; and third, volunteers should be chosen because of a pre-existing criteria. However, it wasn't until 1964, when the World Medical Association published the Declaration of Helsinki, a statement of ethical principles for research on human beings, that informed consent became an ethical principle in research, which included the ability of individuals to refuse to participate, and participants were free to withdraw from the research at any time. The Declaration of Helsinki is not legally binding but informs international laws on research. The latest version was adopted by the World Medical Association in 2013 and will be discussed in the last section of this chapter.

Therefore, the ethical approach to obtaining informed consent from prisoners has focused on developing consent forms which focus on protection from coercion and independence of the research from routine healthcare professionals or prison administration, with the extent and limits of the risks and benefits of participating (Christopher et al., 2017; Pope et al., 2007). However, the process of consent is to support individuals to autonomously decide if they wish to participate in a specific research study. There are many challenges to this approach within a prison setting. The autonomy of prisoners can be considered to be incompatible with prison regimes and legally imposed limitations on their liberty (Gostin et al., 2007). Prisoners may have limited situations in prison in which they are encouraged to make autonomous decisions, and therefore this process may appear alien to them. The consent process within the prison setting needs to focus on the risks and potential benefits for prisoners participating within the confines of a prison setting. For example, regarding confidentiality, if a prisoner participates in a study regarding a new treatment for a certain illness, it may become known by both prison staff and fellow prisoners that the prisoner has this illness.

During the process of informed consent, an essential element is that the prisoner needs to understand the information being presented to them, especially with regard to the prisoner's reading skills. Other considerations include the low level of educational and literacy of prisoners (Moser et al., 2004), high rates of mental illness, learning disabilities, traumatic brain injuries, cognitive impairment, sensory impairment and risk factors which may permanently or temporarily affect cognitive abilities, such as illegal drug use (Binswanger et al., 2009; Binswanger et al., 2012; Maschi et al., 2012; Williams et al., 2010; Fazel et al., 2001). A unique challenge to informed consent may occur for prisoners who have endured prolonged solitary confinement and this has also been shown to have an impact on comprehension (Haney, 2003). Therefore, it is important to consider the reading level of the content of information presented to prisoners and to lower this if necessary to enhance their understanding of content, which has been demonstrated to be effective with older adults (Sugarman et al., 1998; Rikkert et al., 1997). A further approach which has been developed is that of extended conversations, which encourage potential participants to discuss the research and ask questions to gain an understanding of the risks and benefits of participating. One example is that of 'teach-to-goal' consent (Kripalani et al., 2008). This process involves providing information to a potential participant either in writing or verbally, followed by a discussion in which questions are answered, and finally the process of teach-back is implemented to assess the potential participant's comprehension of the research. Teach-back involves asking the potential participant to recall information regarding the study in their own words, which has been considered to be a higher ethical standard of consent and has been suggested that it can be easily incorporated into research occurring in the prison environment (Ahalt et al., 2017).

Coercive prison environment

A further element that affects obtaining informed consent by prisoners is that of the 'inherently coercive' prison environment. Coercion to participate in research or any activity within prison has been described as both direct and indirect pressure. Direct pressure can include pressure from prison staff, when the prisoner believes they will be reprimanded or punished if they do not comply with the prison staff. Whilst indirect pressure is more subtle and involves some benefit to the prisoner, such as the potential to leave their cell more frequently and engage with people from outside the prison (Moser et al., 2004). The 'inherently coercive' prison environment may also be due to prisoners' overwhelming beliefs, rightly or wrongly, that this will be beneficial for them in the future if they cooperate with authorities. Therefore, an element of the coercive prison environment is the power differential between prison staff and prisoners, and this extends to any external agency that enters a prison, including researchers, who must understand this complex dynamics and remain aware of their own potential of power over prisoners (Silva et al., 2017). Such a coercive environment, and whether prisoners experience real or perceived coercive pressures, may further impair their ability to make an informed decision to participate in research (Dugosh et al., 2010).

A study completed by Moser et al. (2004) included an exploration of the degree to which prisoners receiving psychiatric care and healthy controls living in the community were vulnerable to coercion to participate in a research study. The concept of coercion was measured by the development of a questionnaire, the Iowa Coercion Questionnaire (ICQ), and included questions, which explored the participant's reasons for participating in the study. Questions explored both overt and covert forms of exploitation, ranging from being threatened to wanting to give back to society. The results identified that significantly more prisoners compared to health controls living in the community reported possible coercion, which included the desire to appear cooperative, to relieve boredom, to have the opportunity to meet new people and to help others. However, whether these aspects meet the definition of coercion is less clear, but Moser et al. (2004) did demonstrate the types of influence that may occur when recruiting participants in prison and that these may possibly be unavoidable.

Whereas, Dugosh et al. (2010) explored coercion of offenders who identified as substance abusers to participate in research, identified them as a doubly vulnerable population and developed the Coercion Assessment Scale (CAS). Similar to the ICQ, the CAS contained three general types of coercion, that is concerns about repercussions of participation or refusal, pressures related to undue monetary influence and generalised pressures. But unlike the ICQ, the CAS was focused on the types of pressures to participate rather than reasons for participating. The highest form of coercion, which was reported by 50 per cent of participants included a positive response to 'I felt the judge would like it if I entered the study' and 'I felt that entering the study would help my court case'. The results of Dugosh et al. (2010) study demonstrated the invasive nature of coercion with regard to prisoners and offender to participate in research, and the clear need for researchers to ensure this is addressed during the consent process, so these misunderstandings can be addressed.

Confidentiality

An essential element for ethical research is that of confidentiality. It has been suggested that confidentiality within the prison setting for prisons participating in research cannot be ensured. Elements within the prison regime, which will affect confidentiality, include the closed nature of a prison, both the controlled and public nature of movements around the prison and the impact of accompanying prisoners to appointments (Gostin et al., 2007). The risk to confidentiality in the prison setting is not only due to the closed environment but also the pressure from the prison administration or police in the search of information (Silva et al., 2017). However, one of the most debated issues concerning confidentiality of research participants in prison is when researchers should break confidentiality due to concerns regarding the safety of the participant, fellow prisoners and staff, security concerns or illegal activity. Her Majesty's Prison and Probation Service has produced relevant guidance, including an overview of situations where it is necessary for researchers to disclose certain information (HMPPS, 2017). The four main reasons to break confidentiality is due to the disclosure of any of the following:

1   Behaviour that is against prison rules
2   Illegal acts, both previous and planned
3   Behaviour that is harmful to themselves (participant) or others
4   Information which raises concern about terrorist, radicalisation or security issues.

Ethical governance of research in prison

The exploration of ethical governance of research in prison will commence with the pivotal paper defining ethical principles in research, the Declaration of Helsinki (World Medical Association, 2013). The current declaration will briefly be explored, focusing on the elements most poignant to research in prison settings and ethical governance. The following section will explore the process of ethical governance of research in prison in the UK, including the roles of both the Health Research Authorities and the National Research Ethics Service, which is responsible for providing ethical approval for all research involving National Health Service (NHS) patients, including prisoners, and Her Majesty's Prison and Probation Service (HMPPS), National Research Committee, whose approval also has to be obtained for health research occurring in prison settings. The last element will include some practical advice to support readers' understanding of how to obtain all the current necessary ethical approvals to undertake research in a prison setting in England and Wales.

Declaration of Helsinki (2013)

The Declaration of Helsinki was first adopted by the World Medical Association (WMA) in 1964, with amendments agreed in 1975, 1983, 1989, 1996,

2000, 2008 and 2013. The declaration applies to all medical research involving human subjects, including research on identifiable human material and data, and was originally written for physicians, but all healthcare professionals are recommended to adopt these principles. The declaration contains a number of sections including general principles risks, burdens and benefits; vulnerable groups and individuals, scientific requirements and research protocols; research ethics committees; privacy and confidentiality; informed consent; use of placebo; post-trial provisions; research registration and public dissemination of results; and unproven interventions in clinical practice. Although the WMA states that the declaration should be read and applied in full, for this section, elements particularly relevant to prison research will be discussed.

The general principles address an issue identified earlier in this chapter: the fact that there remains a lack of health research in the prison setting and the need for research to support evidence-based healthcare provision for prisoners. Both principles 5 and 13 of the declaration broadly discuss this issue, and need to be considered with regard to the prison setting: 'Medical progress is based on research that ultimately must include studies involving human subject' and 'Groups that are underrepresented in medical research should be provided appropriate access to participation in research'. However, when applying the declaration to research within the prison setting, there is a need to consider how principle 15 of the declaration will be implemented: 'Appropriate compensation and treatment for subjects who are harmed as a result of participating in research must be ensured'. The vulnerable groups and individuals principles clearly state that medical research with this population, which would include prisoners,

> is only justified if the research is responsive to the health needs or priorities of this group and the research cannot be carried out in a non-vulnerable group. In addition, this group should stand to benefit from the knowledge, practices or interventions that result from the research.

The criteria of principle 20 support the development of research with prisoners, which would begin to create evidenced-based physical and mental healthcare for prisoners whilst serving their sentence.

Health Research Authority, National Research Ethics Service

The Health Research Authority (HRA) supports the National Research Ethics Service (NRES) with the implementation of NHS Research Ethics Committees (RECs). Both the HRA and NRES through RECs are involved in providing ethical approval for all medical research involving NHS patients. The aim and objective of the HRA is to protect the rights, safety, dignity and well-being of research participants. Prior to introducing the ethical process of the NRES REC, it is important to highlight that HRA has to date applied a restrictive approach to involving prisoners in research (Charles et al., 2016). Only research directly relating to prisoners' health that can only be conducted in the prison setting is ethically permissible, which is also supported by the Royal College of Physicians (RCP, 2007). Although this is beginning to change, the committees may be influenced by a lack of understanding as they do not regularly review applications that include prisoners. Only 0.7 per cent of research requiring NRES approval involves the inclusion of prisoners (Charles et al., 2016).

The process of applying for ethical approval from HRA, NRES and HMPPS occurs through the online system of the Integrated Research Application System (IRAS). It is important to note that HRA approval and approval from NRES through a REC are two different approvals, although they occur simultaneously through the IRAS system. HRA approval replaces the old method of obtaining approval from the Research and Development (R+D) departments of each NHS Trust involved in the study, which is now coordinated by the HRA. However, supplementary engagement is still required by the researcher with R+D departments to obtain at least an official letter of access or a research passport. HMPPS National Research Ethics Committee (NREC) will also provide a separate approval for any study that is conducted within the prison setting or with offenders, which is also applied for simultaneously through IRAS. A minimum of three approvals (HRA, NRES and HMPPS) need to be sought and gained before the commencement of the study. Depending on the study design, other committees may also need to provide approval, and IRAS captures the information needed for the relevant approvals from the following review bodies:

- Administration of Radioactive Substances Advisory Committee (ARSAC)
- Confidentiality Advisory Group (CAG)
- Gene Therapy Advisory Committee (GTAC)
- Medicines and Healthcare products Regulatory Agency (MHRA)
- Social Care Research Ethics Committee.

The IRAS supports the submission of a research application through one system, so the applicant only has to enter all the relevant information about their research once, and separate forms will then be populated depending on the type of study and the permissions and approvals required. The generic forms will include information required by HRA and NRES, although further information will be requested for research occurring in a prison setting, which will be submitted to HMPPS. However, prior to the submission of an application on IRAS, it is important that the researcher has obtained ethical approval from their own institution, usually a university, which will then become the sponsor of the study. The sponsor of the research is different from the institution that might be funding the research, as the sponsor is legally responsible for the conduct of the study.

Documents also need to be uploaded and submitted within the application on IRAS; a checklist needs to be completed, which includes documents relevant to all types of research so not all are relevant to each study, but include research protocol; letter from statistician; summary CV for the Chief Investigator; participant information sheet; consent form; letters of invitation to participants; GP/consultant information sheet or letter; interview schedule or topic guides; validated questionnaires; non-validated questionnaires; referee's report or other scientific critique; summary, synopsis or flow diagram of protocol information in non-technical language; cover letter on headed paper; organisation information document; non-NHS site assessment form; letter from sponsor; letter from funder; costing template; schedule of events; contract/study agreement; evidence of sponsor's insurance or indemnity; MHRA notice of 'no objection' letter; confirmation of any other regulatory body (not HMMPS at this stage); and laboratory manual and instructions for use of medical devices. Templates for the majority of these documents can be found on the HRA and HMPPS web pages.

Once the application is submitted, it is reviewed by HRA, and simultaneously submitted to a NRES REC and a HMPPS NREC (discussed in the following section) for ethical consideration. The HRA and NRES REC will both consider the study; HRA assesses the governance and the legal compliance of the study and does this through email contact with the researchers. The NRES REC will first identify if this study is suitable for proportionate review (PR) or needs a full review by a REC. A PR supports an accelerated process when studies raise no ethical issues and is completed by email with the researchers. A full review by a REC involves an appointed REC reviewing the study, and the researchers are invited to attend a REC to answer any of the queries raised in this process. RECs are composed of a number of members and for a committee to be quorate, the following members (minimum of seven and maximum of 15) must be present: the chair, or if unavailable the vice-chair or alternative vice-chair, one lay member or a lay plus member, and one expert member. A lay member or lay plus member is someone who is not a registered healthcare professional and whose primary professional interest is not in clinical research. Whereas expert members are those who are registered healthcare professionals, statisticians and others who work within a specialist field in health.

NRES RECs review over 6,000 research applications each year, through RECs in England (65), Scotland (11), Wales (2) and Northern Ireland (2). Each REC is flagged with a certain speciality to support the development of committee members' expertise in a specific method and approach to research involving health data from human beings. The HRA suggests the following flagged committees are available: establishing research databases; research tissue banks; gene therapy or stem cell clinical trials; medical device studies; phase 1 studies in health volunteers; phase 1 studies in patients; qualitative research; research involving adults lacking capacity; research involving children; research involving prisoners or prisons; and social care research. Therefore, when applying for ethical approval from a REC, it is advisable to identify a REC which is flagged with a specialist in the approach applied in your research. However, although this list suggests that there should be a committee flagged for research involving prisoners or prisons at the time of writing and previously, I have not identified a REC flagged with this speciality. The current approach for ethical approval of research in prison settings is the application to HRA, NRES and HMPPS through one online process, and the three bodies simultaneously review the study.

The outcome of both PR and a full review by a REC are communicated to the researcher by email and the possible options include:

- A favourable opinion occurs when the PR or full review at the REC has no concerns or comments regarding the ethics of the study.
- A favourable opinion with conditions occurs when there are minor and specific changes to documents or there remains a need to provide updated insurance documents.
- A provisional opinion occurs when further information or clarification is required from the applicant, which may occur when a member of a research team attends the REC but cannot provide sufficient information to answer all the queries raised by the committee. Once information is received and reviewed, a favourable opinion can be granted.
- An unfavourable decision occurs when studies cannot be implemented in their current form due to ethical concerns. These studies can be revised and resubmitted as a new application. RECs usually provide detailed information of their ethical concerns to support the researcher in developing their study. However, the researchers have the option to appeal and the original submission will be reviewed by a second REC.
- A no opinion can occur when a study has been submitted for a PR, but the members of the PR identify ethical concerns that require a full review by a REC. Therefore, a no opinion will be the opinion of the PR and then a full review will be completed by a REC and their opinion/decision provided to the researchers. Very occasionally a no opinion occurs following a full review by a REC. This only happens in exceptional circumstances where further substantial information is required, or the REC as a collective feel they cannot provide an opinion.

The timeframes for the decisions throughout this process are clearly stated on the HRA and NRES web page and an overview of the process, excluding the possible outcomes of NRES REC, is presented in the flow diagram in the next section. After a favourable opinion by a REC, the researcher needs to provide an annual and final report to the committee. Any amendments to the protocol need to be submitted to the same REC for approval. Before any diversion from the protocol occurs, these are classified as substantial or non-substantial amendments. Substantial amendments include changes to procedures undertaken by participants or changes to the sponsor of the study as the researcher has changed institutions. Non-substantial amendments include changes to the funding arrangements or the research team.

Her Majesty's Prison and Probation Service, National Research Committee

Research occurring in a prison setting or with offenders in the UK will also need to gain ethical permission from Her Majesty's Prison and Probation Service (HMPPS) National Research Committee (NRC). This process addresses three main elements relevant to the prison setting. First, the implications of the research on the operational delivery of the prison. This is a similar consideration to that of R+D departments within NHS Trusts, as it is unlikely that any research occurring in an NHS Trust or a prison setting will not have an impact on the operational delivery of that institution. In the prison setting, extra movements of prisoners to participate in research could affect the operational delivery of the prison by removing prison staff from their normal duties, which could lead to other prisoners spending longer in their cells. Therefore, an important consideration of research in the prison setting is how to conduct the research within the prison regime. An approach for qualitative research could involve interviewing prisoners in private rooms when they are attending work, classes, health clinics or other initiatives, so they do not need to be escorted to meet with the researchers.

Second, the NRC will complete an evaluation of data protection and security and the implications for the prison. Data protection and security is essential in all research, and this is emphasised for the prison population throughout the research process. Elements that need to be considered include the storage of consent forms and how these will be transported to a secure environment if this is within a university and not the prison setting. Audio data is considered as personal identifying information; robust methods for transporting, transcribing and destroying of this identifiable data are required. An important element is the documentation of how disclosure of information regarding a breach of prison security will be addressed. A further element for consideration is the equipment necessary to complete the research, as clearance by the prison will be required. Items allowed into the prison will depend on the level of security of the prison, but items such as audio equipment, phones and laptops will always require clearance.

Third, NRC will assess the relevance of the research for a prison setting and if the research supports the current priorities of the prison service. Priorities are influenced by the Prison and Probation Ombudsman (PPO) who investigates deaths within the prison setting. Recently, there has been a focus on self-inflicted deaths, including those that occur in the early days in custody and segregation, as well as deaths from natural causes with a focus on the healthcare provision, pathways and the use of restraints (PPO, 2017). Prior to this, the PPO (2016) focused on older prisoners and those with dementia, as described in Chapter 4. However, even following approval from HRA, NRES REC and HMPPS NRC, the decision to grant access to a prison ultimately lies with the governor of each individual prison.

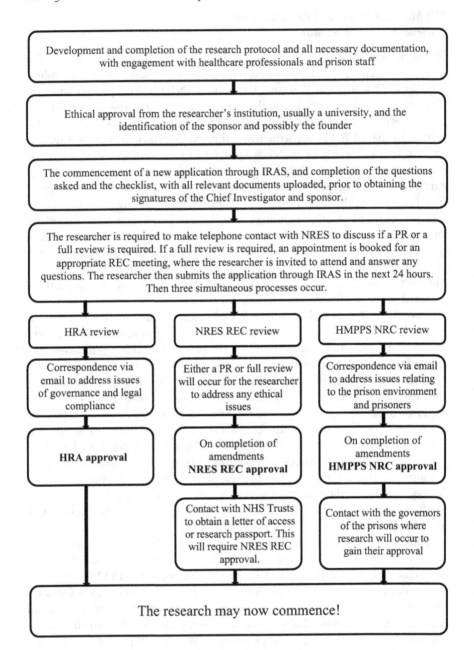

Figure 7.1 Process of obtaining consent for health research within a prison setting

The process for NRC approval is similar to NRES REC. Once data has been entered into IRAS and identified as prison research, information regarding the impact on the operation of the prison, data protection and security and the relevance of the research to current prison priorities will be requested within IRAS. On completion of this element of the application, the IRAS application is complete and the researcher phones the HRA for an appointment for a review of their study. There are clear documented timelines for the process of ethical approval. The NRC will notify the outcome of their review in writing. This committee is selective due to the high volume of applications, although only a few of these are health related. Following a successful outcome, any amendments need to be approved by NRC, such as widening the research to include another prison or increasing the number of participants within one prison. On completion of the study, a summary of results is required by the NRC to enable them to share the findings with the Ministry of Justice and HMPPS. Unsuccessful applications are allowed one further attempt to submit to NRC, however, only if all the reasons for the previous rejection have been completely addressed.

The following is a flow diagram to provide an overview of all the current and necessary ethical approvals to undertake research in a prison setting in the UK.

Summary

This chapter has explored the historical context of research within prison settings, and the research that occurred on prisoners without their understanding or consent, which led to the development of long-term health conditions, sterilisation and death. These acts have supported the development of ethical research practices, which have been informed by the Nuremberg Code, Belmont Report and the Declaration of Helsinki. The practicalities of research within prison include the difficulties of obtaining informed consent within the coercive prison environment, along with challenges of confidentiality. Finally, this chapter explores the necessary ethical approvals that need to be obtained before beginning a research study with prisoners in a prison in England.

References

Advisory Committee on Human Radiation Experiments (1996). *The Human Radiation Experiments*. Oxford: Oxford University Press.

Ahalt, C., Binswanger, I.A., Steinman, M., Tulsky, J., Williams, B.A. (2012). Confined to ignorance: the absence of prisoner information from nationally representative health data sets. *Journal of General Internal Medicine*, 27(2): 160–166.

Ahalt, C., Bolano, M., Wang, E.A., Williams, B. (2015). The state of research funding from the National Institutes of Health for criminal justice health research. *Annals of Internal Medicine*, 162(5): 345–352.

Ahalt, C., Sudore, R., Bolano, M., Metzger, L., Darby, A.M., Williams, B. (2017). "Teach-to-goal" to better assess informed consent comprehension among incarcerated clinical research participants. *AMA Journal of Ethics*, 19(9): 862–872.

Alving, A., Craige, B., Pullman, T., Whorton, M., Jones, R., Eichelberger, L. (1948). Procedures used at Stateville penitentiary for the testing of potential antimalarial agents. *The Journal of Clinical Investigation*, 27(3): 2–5.

Annas, G., Grodin, M. (1992). *The Nazi Doctors and the Nuremberg Code: Human Rights in Human Experimentation*. New York: Oxford University Press.

Appleman, L. (2020). The captive lab rat: human medical experimentation in the carceral state. *Boston College Law Review*, 61(1).

Binswanger, I.A., Krueger, P.M., Steiner, J.F. (2009). Prevalence of chronic medical conditions among jail and prison inmates in the USA compared with the general population. *Journal of Epidemiology and Community Health*, 63(11): 912–919.

Binswanger, I.A., Redmond, N., Steiner, J.F., Hicks, L.S. (2012). Health disparities and the criminal justice system: an agenda for further research and action. *Journal of Urban Health*, 89(1): 98–107.

Boly, W. (1977). The Heller experiments. *Oregon Times Magazine*, November, 45.

Chancellor, J.C., Blue, R.S., Cengel, K.A., Auñón-Chancellor, S.M., Rubins, K.H., Katzgraber, H.G., Kennedy, A.R. (2018). Limitations in predicting the space radiation health risk for exploration astronauts. *Microgravity*, 4: 8.

Charles, A., Draper, H. (2012). Equivalence of care in prison medicine: is equivalence of process the right measure of equity? *Journal of Medical Ethics*, 38(4): 215–218.

Charles, A., Rid, A., Davies, H., Draper, H. (2016). Prisoners as research participants: current practice and attitudes in the UK. *Journal of Medical Ethics*, 42: 246–252.

Christopher, P.P., Candilis, P.J., Rich, J.D., Lidz, C.W. (2011). An empirical ethics agenda for psychiatric research involving prisoners. *AJOB Primary Research*, 2(4): 18–25.

Christopher, P.P., Garcia-Sampson, L.G., Stein, M., Johnson, J., Rich, J., Lidz, C. (2017). Enrolling in clinical research while incarcerated: what influences participants' decisions. *The Hastings Center Report*, 47(2): 21–29.

Christopher, P.P., Stein, M.D., Johnson, J.E., Rich, J.D., Friedmann, P.D., Clarke, J.G., Lidz, C.W. (2016). Exploitation of prisoners in clinical research: perceptions of study participants. *IRB Ethics and Human Research*, 38(1): 7–12.

Cislo, A.M., Trestman, R. (2013). Challenges and solutions for conducting research in correctional settings: the US experience. *International Journal of Law and Psychiatry*, 36: 304–310.

Council of Europe (2005). *Additional Protocol to the Convention on Human Rights and Biomedicine, Concerning Biomedical Research*. Available from: http://conventions.coe.int/Treaty/EN/Treaties/Html/195.htm [Accessed on: 24 May 2020].

DHEW Report (1976). *Report and Recommendations: Research Involving Prisoners* (pp. 76–131). Washington, DC: US Department of Health, Education and Welfare, No. (OS).

Dugosh, K.L., Festinger, D.S., Croft, J.R., Marlowe, D.B. (2010). Measuring coercion to participate in research within a doubly vulnerable population: initial development of the coercion assessment scale. *Journal of Empirical Research on Human Research Ethics*, 5(1): 93–102.

Emanuel, E. (2008). Addressing exploitation: reasonable availability versus fair benefits. In J.S. Hawkins, E.J. Emanuel (Eds.) *Exploitation and Developing Countries: The Ethics of Clinical Research* (pp. 63–104). Princeton, NJ: Princeton University Press.

Fazel, S., Hope, T., O'Donnell, I., Jacoby, R. (2001). Hidden psychiatric morbidity in elderly prisoners. *The British Journal of Psychiatry*, 179: 535–539.

Fitzpatrick, F. (2012). *The Prisoner's Dilemma: The History, Ethical Dimensions, and Evolving Regulatory Landscape of Clinical Trials on Inmates.* Cambridge: Harvard University Press.

Goldberger, J., Wheeler, G. (1915). Experimental pellagra in the human subject brought about by a restricted diet. *Public Health Report,* 30: 3336.

Gostin, L., Vanchieri, C., Pope, A. (2007). *Institute of Medicine (US) Committee on Ethical Considerations for Revisions to DHHS Regulations for Protection of Prisoners Involved in Research. Ethical Considerations for Research Involving Prisoners.* Washington, DC: National Academies Press.

Haney, C. (2003). Mental health issues in long-term solitary and "supermax" confinement. *Crime and Delinquency,* 49(1): 124–156.

Heller, C. (1963). Pacific Northwest Research Foundation, proposal for Atomic Energy Commission, Division of Biology and Medicine. "Effects of ionizing radiation on the testicular function of man" (ACHRE No. DOE-122994-A-2).

Her Majesty's Prison and Probation Service (2017). *Application Guidance.* Available from: www.gov.uk/government/organisations/her-majestys-prison-and-probation-service/about/research#further-information [Accessed on: 24 May 2020].

Hoffman, S. (2000). Beneficial and unusual punishment: an argument in support of prisoner participation in clinical trials. *Indiana Law Review,* 33(2): 475–515.

Hornblum, A. (1998). *Acres of Skin: Human Experiments at Holmesburg Prison.* New York: Routledge.

Ivy, A.C. (1948). Ethics governing the service of prisoners as subjects as medical experiments. Report of a committee appointed by the Governor Dwight H. Green of Illinois. *Journal of the American Association,* 136: 457–458.

Kouyoumdjian, F.G., McIsaac, K.E., Liauw, J., Green, S., Karachiwalla, F., Siu, W., Burkholder, K., Binswanger, I., Kiefer, L., Kinner, S.A., Korchinski, M., Matheson, F.I., Young, P., Hwang, S.W. (2015). A systematic review of randomized controlled trials of interventions to improve the health of persons during imprisonment and in the year after release. *American Journal of Public Health,* 105(4): e13–e33.

Kouyoumdjian, F.G., Schuler, A., Hwang, S.W., Matheson, F.I. (2015b). Research on the health of people who experience detention or incarceration in Canada: a scoping review. *BMC Public Health,* 15(1): 1.

Kripalani, S., Bengtzen, R., Henderson, L.E., Jacobson, T.A. (2008). Clinical research in low-literacy populations: using teach-back to assess comprehension of informed consent and privacy information. *IRB,* 30(2): 13–19.

Langer, E. (1964). Human experimentation: cancer studies at Sloan-Kettering stir public debate on medical ethics. *Science,* 143(3606): 551–553.

Lederer, S. (1995). *Subjected to Science: Human Experimentation in America Before the Second World War.* Baltimore, MD: John Hopkins University Press.

Marini, J., Sheard, M., Bridges, I. (1976). An evaluation of "informed consent" with volunteer prisoner subjects. *The Yale Journal of Biology and Medicine,* 49(5): 427–437.

Maschi, T., Kwak, J., Ko, E., Morrissey, M.B. (2012). Forget me not: dementia in prison. *Gerontologist,* 52(4): 441–451.

Moreno, J. (1997). Reassessing the influence of the Nuremberg code on American medical ethics. *Journal of Contemporary Health Law Policy,* 13: 347–360.

Moser, D.J., Arndt, S., Kanz, J., Benjamin, M.L., Bayless, J.D., Akcakaya, R.L.R., Paulsen, J.S., Flaum, M. (2004). Coercion and informed consent in research involving prisoners. *Comprehensive Psychiatry,* 45(1): 1–9.

Newman, L. (2005). Maurice Hilleman. *British Medical Journal,* 330(7498): 1028.

Nuremberg Code (1947). In A. Mischerlich, F. Mielke (Eds.) *Doctors of Infamy: The Story of the Nazi Medical Crimes* (pp. xxiii–xxv). New York: Schuman.

Office for Human Research Protections (1979). *The Belmont Report. US Department of Health and Human Services. Regulations and Policy.* Available from: www.hhs.gov/ohrp/regula tions-and-policy/belmont-report/index.html [Accessed on: 24 May 2020].

Pappworth, M. (1967). *Human Guinea Pigs: Experimentation on Man.* London: Routledge.

Pope, A., Vanchieri, C., Gostin, L.O. (2007). *Ethical Considerations for Research Involving Prisoners.* Washington, DC: National Academies Press.

Prison and Probation Ombudsman (PPO) (2016). Learning Lessons Bulletin. Fatal Incidents Investigations. Issue 11. Dementia. London, UK.

Prison and Probation Ombudsman (PPO) (2017). Learning Lessons Bulletin. Fatal Incidents Investigations. Issue 13. Self-inflected deaths. London, UK.

Reiter, K. (2009). Experimentation on prisoners: persistent dilemmas in rights and regulations. *California Law Review*, 97: 501–566.

Rikkert, M.B., van den Bercken, J.H., ten Have, H.A., Hoefnagels, W.H. (1997). Experienced consent in geriatrics research: a new method to optimise the capacity to consent in frail elderly subjects. *Journal of Medical Ethics*, 23(5): 271–276.

Royal College of Physicians (2007). *Guidelines on the Practice of Ethics Committees in Medical Research with Human Participants.* Available from: http://bookshop.rcplondon.ac.uk/con tents/pub232-e0da0967-8bed-4ac3-a12f-b05ad6a6c873.pdf [Accessed on: 24 May 2020].

Silva, D.S., Matheson, F.I., Lavery, J.V. (2017). Ethics of health research with prisoners in Canada. *BMC Medical Ethics*, 18: 31.

Smoyer, A., Blankenship, K., Belt, B. (2009). Compensation for incarcerated research participants: diverse state policies suggest a new research agenda. *American Journal of Public Health*, 99(10): 1746–1752.

Stanley, L.L. (1922). Analysis of one thousand testicular substance implantations. *Endocrinology*, 6: 787–788.

Sugarman, J., McCrory, D.C., Hubal, R.C. (1998). Getting meaningful informed consent from older adults: a structured literature review of empirical research. *Journal of American Geriatric Society*, 46(4): 517–524.

Weindling, P. (2001). The origins of informed consent: the International Scientific Commission on Medical War Crimes, and the Nuremberg code. *Bulletin of the History of Medicine*, 75(1): 37–71.

Wertheimer, A. (1999). *Exploitation.* Princeton, NJ: Princeton University Press.

Williams, B.A., McGuire, J., Lindsay, R.G., et al. (2010). Coming home: health status and homelessness risk of older pre-release prisoners. *Journal of General Internal Medicine*, 25(10): 1038–1044.

World Medical Association (1964). *WMA Declaration of Helsinki – Ethical Principles for Medical Research Involving Human Subjects.* Available from: www.wma.net/wp-content/uploads/2018/07/DoH-Jun1964.pdf [Accessed on: 24 May 2020].

World Medical Association (2013). WMA declaration of Helsinki – ethical principles for medical research involving human subjects. *JAMA*, 310(20): 2191–2194.

8 Ethical framework for research in prison

Joanne Brooke

Biomedical ethics in prison research

The four pillars of biomedical ethics have been widely explored in healthcare research and embedded into guidelines and policies. The four pillars, of which none is more important than the other, include autonomy, beneficence, non-maleficence, and justice (Beauchamp and Childress, 2001). They have been explained in Chapter 6 and will now be applied to conducting research in a prison setting. The discussion under each pillar will include prison research with participants who are prisoners, but also prison staff, and health and social care staff.

Autonomy

The aspects of autonomy will be discussed with regard to prison research and these include respect for autonomy, confidentiality and autonomy, protection and autonomy, and perceived choice and autonomy. A researcher will need to consider all of these aspects to inform the development of their research, especially methods of recruitment and the identification of when breaking confidentiality may need to occur, and ultimately the positive and negative impact on prisoners of their research.

Respect for autonomy

The respect of prisoner's autonomy has been suggested as an important element in improving public health within a prison setting, which is enabled by the implementation of social science research (Shaw and Elger, 2015). Traditionally, medical research in prison has focused on the prevalence of infectious diseases such as HIV, hepatitis B and C (Weild et al., 2000) and tuberculosis (Coninx et al., 2000), and the risks for and prevalence of chronic medical conditions (Binswanger et al., 2009; Herbert et al., 2012), with the aim to understand the treatment needs of prisoners and to ensure equivalence of access to healthcare. Medical research in prison is important, although it may not address the individual health needs of prisoners and identify specific aspects of their healthcare needs that are not being met. However, social science research could address this issue through qualitative research with prisoners, which may identify gaps in healthcare that could be addressed, whilst maintaining the confidentiality of the prisoners and the researcher implementing steps to improve their healthcare. Shaw and Elger (2015) suggest that social science research within the prison setting can support and benefit both prisoners and prison staff through six processes:

First, social science research may include semi-structured interviews or focus groups with prisoners. This approach may support prisoners to discuss their personal experience and highlight issues they have experienced with both the provision and receipt of healthcare. Respecting prisoner's autonomy will occur through empowering prisoners to talk and share their experiences in a safe and confidential space. However, social science research that adopts this approach without the intention of recommending and supporting changes to healthcare services may be harmful to prisoners. The outcome and the influence of the research is essential for prisoners, as this may be the first time their concerns have been listened to and taken seriously with due respect to their autonomy. Therefore, it could be argued social science research that does not intend to support change following qualitative data collection does not respect the autonomy of prisoners, as the research did not provide the participating prisoners with the ability to be autonomous and affect their environment (Shaw and Elger, 2015).

Second, a consequence of the research may include positive changes to the prison environment and/or healthcare provision for the prisoner. It is important this process occurs through maintaining and respecting the autonomy of the participating prisoners (Shaw and Elger, 2015). Through this process, prisoners will experience improved self-esteem as their experiences and concerns were taken seriously, and this can be further developed by engaging prisoners in participatory research supporting them to be peer researchers (Martin et al., 2008).

Third, once prisoners begin to see the changes to their environment and healthcare provision because of their participation in research, Shaw and Elger (2015) suggest that prisoners are likely to also feel respected by the prison administration and prison staff, as their thoughts and opinions influenced the solution and change to the provision of healthcare.

Fourth, if prisoners feel their autonomy is being respected by prison administration and prison staff, this may decrease their aggression towards prison staff and possibly other prisoners (Shaw and Elger, 2015). This has previously been demonstrated through sociotherapy programmes within mental healthcare provision for prisoners, where prison staff are respectful partners, to break down the 'them and us' attitude of both prison staff and prisoners (de Montmollin, 1985).

Fifth, prison staff would benefit from increased respect from prisoners and a reduction of the risk of aggression towards them (Shaw and Elger, 2015). Aggression directed at prison staff from prisoners is a complex phenomenon and often associated with the age and aggressive nature of the prisoner, but also the prison environment (Lahm, 2009), both of which might be addressed through the respect of a prisoner's autonomy.

Sixth, prisoners would also benefit from increased respect from prison staff (Shaw and Elger, 2015). Increased respect for prisoners by prison staff may occur due to the change in prisoner's behaviour. For example prison staff have been involved in the support of prisoners with mental health difficulties through building a foundation of mutual respect and ongoing communication and cooperation (Applebaum et al., 2001).

Finally, increased mutual respect between prison staff and prisoners would support the raising of issues by prisoners to prison staff, and vice versa, without the need for the intervention of social science research (Shaw and Elger, 2015).

Confidentiality and autonomy

The impact of confidentiality has been discussed with regard to autonomy of participants in Chapter 7 and the complex issue of maintaining confidentiality of research participants in the closed environment of a prison setting (Giordano et al., 2007). The confidentiality of participants is paramount unless the participant provides information that is of concern, such as behaviour that is against prison rules, illegal acts, behaviour that is harmful to themselves or others or information that raises concern regarding security. The role of the researcher is to understand when confidentiality may need to breached, such as the need to report any increased risk of self-harm to the member of prison staff who is responsible for the prisoner's Assessment Care in Custody and Teamwork (ACCT) for clear documentation and an action plan (Ward and Bailey, 2012). Therefore, there is a need to balance confidentiality between prison service obligations of duty of care and developing a research relationship with participants. Prisoners as participants need to be aware of how and when confidentiality will be broken, and therefore absolute confidentiality cannot be guaranteed. This has been referred to as 'limited confidentiality' within research in the prison setting (Cowburn, 2005). The limited confidentiality of participants in prison research commences with the process of recruitment, as a member of the prison or healthcare staff will need to identify prisoners who meet the inclusion and exclusion criteria for each study. This needs to be recognised and discussed with potential participants during recruitment (Schlosser, 2008).

Protection and autonomy

Prisoners have been protected from being subjected to research since the World Medical Association adopted the Declaration of Helsinki (1964). However, when does the ethical consideration of protection of vulnerable populations begin to affect their autonomy (Spencer, 2017)? The protection of vulnerable populations, such as prisoners, prevents individuals classified as vulnerable from having the same opportunity as others to participate in research, affecting their autonomy (Liabo et al., 2017). This element will also be considered later, as equal and equitable access to research aims to ensure the ethical principle of justice. Vulnerable populations who are not involved in research will gradually become invisible, and other people will begin to make decisions which directly have an impact on them, without them being involved, again affecting their autonomy (Daley, 2015). Therefore, the protection of prisoners against being subjected to research supports their autonomy, but when the protection prevents them from participating due to being a prisoner, then protection is impeding their autonomy.

Perceived afforded choice and autonomy

The importance of autonomy and perceived afforded choice has been explored as components of the self-determination theory (Ryan and Deci, 2000). Autonomy and perceived choice are essential elements of well-being, and within the prison setting, the limitation of both of these concepts may have an impact on the psychological well-being of prisoners (van de Kaap-Deeder et al., 2017). The perception of autonomy and perceived choice by prisoners may differ considerably depending on their personal experience, such as autonomous decisions regarding healthcare (Andorno et al., 2015). The involvement of prisoners in research may improve their perceived provision of choice, and indirectly their satisfaction with autonomy, which may support their psychological well-being. A study involving Belgium prisoners identified enhancing perceived choice and autonomy satisfaction can support and improve prisoners' quality of life (van de Kaap-Deeder et al., 2017). Therefore, the lack of or provision of autonomy provided to prisoners is beyond an ethical concern within research, but one which affects prisoners' physical and mental health.

Beneficence – the duty to 'do good'

Beneficence and non-maleficence are two principles which focus on the analysis of risk and will be separated in this discussion. Beneficence is the focus on the benefit element of the risk analysis and the potential benefits of the research. Beneficence is supported in research as described earlier, as prisoners may benefit from being listened to by social researchers and their involvement in problem-solving some of the issues they identified. The term that has now been applied to this research is prison research from 'inside-out' (Thrasher et al., 2019). This approach originated from the Inside-Out Prison Exchange Program, developed by Lori Pompa, and the teaching of courses within the prison setting with prisoners and external students (King et al., 2019). This had been developed and implemented in many countries in many formats, such as prisoners and undergraduate social work students (Smoyer, 2019) and within prisons in England. This approach has been applied to address students' own prejudices by exploring their beliefs and attitudes whilst studying with prisoners (King et al., 2019). The concept of inside-out is both an exchange and an engagement between people inside the prison and outside of the prison to develop equality and equity as though the walls of the prison did not exist (Thrasher et al., 2019). The principle of beneficence can be addressed through research that adopts the ethos of the inside-out approach, to engage with prisoners as participants, with research that will eventually benefit them, either physically or psychologically through being listened to, heard and being involved in the development of a solution.

An example of this research approach explored the synthetic cannabinoid markets in a prison in England (Ralphs et al., 2017). The research was commissioned because of the growth of seizures by prison staff of synthetic cannabinoids (spice) and an increased number of incidents believed to be related to these substances. Data was collected through ethnographic principles to understand the whole prison environment, which included data on drug seizures, observations and analysis of bodycams when prison staff were dealing with drug-related incidents and workshops where prison staff and prisoners discussed their experiences. Following the collection of this data, interviews and focus groups were conducted separately with prison staff and prisoners. This included seven semi-structured interviews with prisoners and four focus groups with 20 prisoners. The contribution from prisoners who had been involved with drugs was invaluable to this study, without whom the true depth and understanding of the issue would not have become apparent. The involvement of prisoners willing to discuss their drug habits informed realistic recommendations that concentrated on the reduction of the availability and use of synthetic cannabinoids in prison rather than on an unrealistic aim of striving for a drug-free prison.

Non-maleficence – the duty to 'not do bad'

Non-maleficence is the focus on the deficit or cost element of risk analysis and the potential harm of the research. This discussion will focus on social research within prison settings, rather than the risk analysis of medical trials. An important element within this ethical approach is the possible harm that may occur when information obtained through the research process may need to be disclosed to prison administration because of the risk to the individual participant, to others or to the security of the prison. The ethical approach to research is to inform participants of the possibility of a breach of confidentiality if certain information is disclosed, with an explanation of what constitutes information that raises concerns. However, research exploring prisoners' participation in social science research identified that prisoners did not experience any harm (Copes et al., 2012).

Psychological harms for prisoners participating in research must also be considered, especially when studies focus on events and experiences that may be distressing for participants. The recalling and discussion of these events through semi-structured interviews may increase participants' stress and affect their mood negatively. Evidence from community-dwelling participants suggests although this form of research may cause stress, it does not lead to adverse events (Labott et al., 2013). However, the added vulnerability of prisoners needs to be considered and appropriate support should be made available if a participant becomes distressed during or after a research interview.

A further psychological harm that is not always identified or acknowledged is the harm that occurs on completion of social science research. The prisoner may have had extra time outside of the cell to participate in the research and engage socially with a researcher who was interested in listening to and understanding their experiences. Therefore, it has been recognised that feelings of loss and sadness can occur on the completion of study for both participants and researchers (Abbott and Scott, 2019). This highlights the need for closing the study through ethically closing relationships with participants and a safe exit through reducing participants' sense of loss and possible abandonment, which needs to be planned as carefully as all other elements of a research study (Abbott and Scott, 2019).

Justice

The ethical pillar of justice is to treat all people fairly, equally and equitably. Within research the aim is to ensure benefits, and possible burdens and harms are shared equitably across groups or arms of a research study. All research should ensure no group is exploited (Macklin, 2014). This is especially important with research in the prison setting, as exploitation can occur through recruitment and as participants should not be included just because they are a convenient population. The development of explicit inclusion and exclusion criteria needs to be developed and implemented to ensure equal opportunities for participants (Macklin, 2014). However, there remains a need to reduce the inequity of healthcare provision in prison settings, and excluding research with prisoners could be considered an act of injustice, as they can make significant contributions (Spencer et al., 2017).

Development of an ethical protocol for prison research

The ethics of research with prisoners extends beyond traditional research ethics involving human subjects. Therefore, this element will build on the four pillars of biomedical ethics and develop them to address particular challenges of ethical research within the closed environment of a prison. The ethics of research and prison research have been discussed in previous chapters, and there is a wealth of information available to understand ethics in research. The first section in this chapter will guide and support researchers to develop an ethical protocol for health and social care research, which will support the considerations of an ethical approach at all stages of developing a study occurring in a prison environment. The framework for the development of an ethical protocol will address the four pillars simultaneously through a discussion of how to develop a research proposal for a study within the prison environment. The conclusion of this section will include an overview of the framework in Table 9.1 to support a clear understanding of the theoretical issues being addressed in relation to prison research.

A framework for the development of an ethical protocol for prison research

The framework for the development of an ethical protocol for prison research contains the majority of the structure of the NHS Health Research Authority's template for a protocol of a qualitative study, last updated on 19 March 2018. This structure supports a framework which has been developed to address the four pillars of biomedical ethics at each stage of developing a research proposal for a study within a prison setting. However, it is acknowledged that this structure is primarily for qualitative research and may need to be amended to address the specific requirements of different institutions and regulatory bodies across different countries. Therefore, this framework is a guide to support researchers to apply ethical considerations during the development and construction of their prison research. Some mandatory elements of a protocol have not been included as they are factual elements that need to be completed for all research and are not specific for the development of research in a prison setting.

1 Rationale

An ethical rationale for research especially one that is conducted in a prison environment must fully explain why this research is important. This will include links to relevant prison policies and current issues, whilst considering prisoners as a vulnerable population because of the nature of previous abusive prison research. These components must be addressed alongside the justification and social validity of the research. Her Majesty's Prison and Probation Service (HMPPS) and governors of individual prisons in England and Wales are unlikely to provide ethical or access approvals for research that does not meet their current specific aims and objectives to improve health and social care for prisoners. Therefore, the emphasis is on the researcher to understand and include contemporary government, national and regional discussions and published papers.

The rationale needs to address the social validity and justification of the research, which has often been assessed by answering the question 'so what?' to support the understanding of the impact of research on both participants and the wider society (Wester, 2011). Research with social validity can address the two principles of justice, equity and equality of access and provision of gold-standard healthcare. A further element of equality which will be addressed is that prisoners should have equal opportunities as the general public to participate in ethically conducted research (Ahalt et al., 2017). Social validity has been developed within behavioural sciences to ensure behavioural interventions were relevant and appropriate to patients and sustainable in the community, and originates from the work of Wolf (1978) and Kazdin (1977). A framework to assess social validity was developed by Wolf (1978), which assesses the social importance of behavioural science interventions, but this approach of exploring goals, procedures and effects can be applied to research within a prison setting. The social validity of a study can be developed through engagement with stakeholders and people with the characteristics of the potential participants, referred to as patient and public involvement (Bagley et al., 2016), which will be discussed in more depth in section 9.2.

2 Theoretical framework

The theoretical framework of the research needs to provide a clear explanation of why this approach will address the problem identified and an overview of this approach. A theoretical framework is essential in prison research because of the historical context of research in prisons. The inclusion of a theoretical framework supports the reliability and validity of research and the ethical principle of beneficence as recommendations from robust research support positive changes to practice to meet the health and social care needs of prisoners. The reliability and validity of the research are supported through the implementation of a theoretical framework by four principles.

First, the presentation of theoretical assumptions allows the reader to understand the researcher's theoretical assumptions. Second, theoretical frameworks enable the researcher to connect to existing knowledge, and this provides evidence for the choice of methods to answer the problem identified. Third, a theoretical framework should enable the researcher to progress from simply describing the problem identified or phenomenon to critically discussing the various aspects of the phenomenon. Lastly, a theoretical framework or theory will prevent the researcher from overgeneralising their results and provide a structure on how to discuss the relevance of the key findings and how these may differ in different circumstances. For example, in research in prisons in England and Wales, the security category of the prison needs to be considered, as the results of research conducted in an open prison may not be the same or possibly relevant to a maximum security prison, and therefore the results cannot be generalised without recognition of the differences.

3 Aims, objectives and outcomes

The aims, objectives and outcomes need to align with the rationale and theoretical framework for the research, whilst applying a neutral approach and addressing the needs identified by the prison administration. Furthermore, prior to the writing of the aims, objectives and outcomes, consideration of the topic under investigation needs to ensure the focus of the research does not incidentally explore information that may include unprosecuted criminal activity or activity that might affect the security of the prison.

4 Study design

The study design of the research should be clearly stated and support both the rationale and theoretical framework. There are four major types of qualitative research design: phenomenology, ethnography, grounded theory and case study (which can also be applied in quantitative research designs). Phenomenological research is the study of experience, sometimes referred to as 'lived experience'. Prominent phenomenological philosophers, such as Husserl, Heidegger, Merleau-Ponty and Sartre, have influenced a number of phenomenological research approaches, which all include in-depth interviews or focus groups with participants (Smith et al., 2009). Ethnography is the study of individual cultures. There are many forms of this approach including confessional ethnography and autoethnography, although overwhelmingly ethnographical research focuses on the observation of social practices and interactions. Grounded theory originally developed by Glaser and Strauss (1967) is a form of qualitative research which supports a process to data collection which is flexible and informs the development of a theory. Methods of data collection can include interviews, focus groups and observations. Each of these qualitative designs is appropriate for the prison setting, although some may be more difficult to implement than others, such as observations of the phenomenon under exploration.

5 Methods of data collection and data analysis

Data collection methods need to be described in detail. This is particularly pertinent for research in the prison setting. Each method of data collection needs to be carefully considered with regard to data collection through observations. Four elements need to be specifically applied to the prison environment.

First, what will be observed and will this include anybody within the prison environment who has not specifically provided informed consent to be observed, which would be a breach of their autonomy and possibly cause of harm, non-maleficence?

Second, how will the observation be documented? If the observation is to be recorded, what equipment is required and will the prison administration allow this equipment into the prison, and if so how will the equipment and recording be protected?

Third, who will complete the observing? Will they have the skills and understanding to react to different scenarios that may occur within a prison setting?

Fourth, will the observation of the phenomenon affect the prison regime? What are the implications of the observations on prison staff and the on completion of their duties?

Both interviews and focus group discussions need to consider the guide for discussions and how this is developed, but with reference to the prison setting. The considerations are similar to those of observations, including who will be conducting the interviews and how these will be recorded. An important consideration is the involvement of prison officers to support the movement of prisoners to participate in the research, as this additional duty can negatively affect the prison regime and specifically other prisoners (non-participants) who may be up locked in their cell during scheduled recreation (Brooke and Rybacka, 2020).

Methods of data analysis are equally as important to and align with the qualitative design of the research and the method of data collection. Data analysis of transcripts of audio recorded interviews and focus groups may occur through a number of different approaches such as framework analysis (Gale et al., 2013), interpretative phenomenological analysis (Smith et al., 2009) or thematic analysis (Braun and Clarke, 2006). Each of these approaches needs to be clearly explained, including who is transcribing the data, and if this is outsourced, how will the confidentiality of the participants and elements of prison security be ensured and maintained. A further element relevant to the prison setting is the transfer of data from the prison to the institution where the data will be transcribed, de-identified, analysed and archived, which needs to be within the guidelines of data protection. In the England and Wales, data protection must adhere to the eight principles of the Data Protection Act 2018, which include the storage of data that is fair and lawful, specific for its purpose, adequate and only for what is needed, accurate and up to date, not kept longer than needed, take into account people's rights, kept safe and secure and not transferred outside of the European Economic Area, which are essential to respect the autonomy of research participants.

6 Study setting

Research occurring in a prison setting needs to clearly state and justify why this research needs to occur in this setting. Elements that need to be addressed are where and how the researcher will access prisoners, which as suggested previously needs careful consideration. There is the possibility of accessing participants within the prison setting whilst they are out of the cells and completing other activities. This approach would prevent prison staff being involved in the movement of prisoners. However, this section focuses on the appropriateness of the setting to address the aims of the research, which needs to include specific references to why the research is essential to involve prisoners or prison staff or healthcare professionals working in the prison. The ethical consideration is whether this research can be completed with members of the general public living in the community or whether the research is specific to and can only occur in the prison setting.

7 Sample and eligibility criteria

The eligibility criteria of the sample define the study population and precise definitions of participants who are eligible for the study, including both inclusion and exclusion criteria. Within health and social care research, the definition of participants may include gender, age, socio-economic status and ethnicity but also the clinical condition or disability under study. A number of these variables are self-explanatory in prison research, as prisons are segregated by gender, although there remains limited research on female prisoners, which needs to be addressed (Thomson et al., 2019). Ethnicity is an important variable in prison research, as it has previously been acknowledged that black people make up around 3 per cent of the general population but account for 12 per cent of adult prisoners in England and Wales (The Lammy Review, 2017). Therefore, consideration of how to be inclusive in prison research is essential to respect all prisoners' autonomy. Exclusion criteria are usually dependent on the inclusion criteria. For example an inclusion criterion may be sentenced prisoner only, therefore, prisoners on remand would be an exclusion criterion. However, the choice of inclusion and exclusion criteria will affect both recruitment and attrition of the research.

7.1 SAMPLING, SAMPLE SIZE AND SAMPLING TECHNIQUE

Sampling identifies the number of participants the researcher intends to recruit and the technique used to identify prisoners who meet the inclusion and exclusion criteria. The number of participants depends to some degree on the qualitative research method applied, and recommendations range from 5 to 50 participants (Dworkin, 2012). The important concept in qualitative research data is saturation, and this occurs when interviews with new participants fail to identify new concepts (Mason, 2010). The identification of prisons can occur through a number of recognised and validated methods, including convenience sampling, purposive sampling, a snowball approach or at random. Convenience sampling is a method which collects data from a population who are conveniently available to participate in the study. Purposive sampling applies the judgement of the researcher in selecting participants who meet the purpose of their study, such as the exploration of a particular illness. Within the prison research, convenience sampling would be appropriate to explore prisoners' experience of prison; however, purposive sampling would be appropriate to explore older prisoners' experience of prison. Snowball sampling identifies one or two people who are eligible to participate in the research, and then identifies other people with the same characteristics from their network. Although this approach could work in a prison setting, it is not necessary for the majority of research in closed environments. An element of sampling that is important in the prison setting is to ensure all eligible prisoners have the opportunity to participate if they wish to do so, which leads on to recruitment processes.

8 Recruitment

The recruitment of participants needs to address a number of concepts, which will be discussed individually and with regard to the prison setting. The main challenge is who will identify the potential participants and what method they will use. This is an important consideration in research with prisoners as the researcher is unlikely to have access to identify potential participants and will need to rely on either prison staff or healthcare professionals, which may introduce an element of bias. Researchers who are not members of the healthcare team are not permitted to access health and social care records prior to a potential participant providing consent. Therefore, both prison staff and healthcare professionals may suggest prisoners who they believe to be eligible, rather than apply a systematic approach. Ideally, all prisoners will be provided with a participant information sheet or leaflet, which will identify the purpose of the study as well as inclusion and exclusion criteria. Prisoners can then make an autonomous decision if they wish to participate in the research, which can be expressed through contacting staff, researchers or attending an interview or focus group. This method avoids screening of potential participants by prison staff, administrators or healthcare professionals. A prisoner may pose a potential risk to the researcher, so it is important in the process of recruiting that prison staff and healthcare professionals provide the necessary support (Abbott and Scott, 2018). However, all processes involving prison staff and healthcare professionals supporting the research will be an extra duty and possible burden on their time, and therefore should be kept to a minimum.

8.1 INFORMED CONSENT AND CONFIDENTIALITY

The process of obtaining informed consent from prisoners to participate in research within a coercive prisoner environment has been discussed in depth in Chapter 7. This section will highlight the information that needs to be included in this section of the research protocol. The process of gaining informed consent needs to be explicitly described including discussions with the potential participant regarding the aims and objectives of the research, and the possible associated risks of participating; the provision of written information to potential participants, usually in the form of participant information sheets, which have been reviewed and approved by research ethic committees, regulatory bodies and the prison administration; potential participants have been provided with time to ask questions and have them answered; and the process for identifying potential participants who have the capacity to provide informed consent. The assessment of a prisoner's capacity to consent to participate in research needs to be completed by a researcher or healthcare professional competent to do so. This process includes discussing the research with a potential participant and assessing if they:

1 understand the information relevant to the decision
2 can retain the information
3 use or weigh the information
4 can communicate their decision (by any means).

If a potential participant cannot complete all four of these steps, they are unable to provide informed consent to participate in the research, which has been explained to them. In England and Wales, the Mental Capacity Act 2005 (updated in 2007) provides the legislation and a comprehensive framework for decision making for adults who lack capacity as well as the assumptions of capacity and how to assess capacity. Within the prison setting, it is important to remember the possible variables which may permanently or temporarily affect a prisoner's potential to provide informed consent.

9 Research Ethics Committee and other regulatory reviews and reports

The process of obtaining the necessary approvals for health research within a prison have been presented in detail in Chapter 7, including ethical approval from the researcher's own institution, followed by Health Research Authority, National Research Ethics Service and Her Majesty's Prison and Probation Service approval (please refer to Chapter 7).

9.1 ASSESSMENT OF RISK

The assessment of risk involves both concepts of beneficence and non-maleficence, and because of the historical context of prison research, there is a strong emphasis on minimising the risk to prisoners with a focus on the benefits. This is reflected in the Belmont Report (1979), which stated 'the risk and benefits must be balanced and shown to be in a favourable ration'. However, the Council of Europe (2005) identified that 'non-beneficial' research may include prisoners, but only if the research can only be conducted with prisoners, the outcome will benefit prisoners and the risk to prisoners who do participate is no more than minimal. Therefore, within the research protocol there needs to be a clear analysis of the potential risks and benefits. The risk analysis needs to identify a risk management plan to deal with any potential risk or harm to a participant. This plan also needs to include the mechanisms for safeguarding, and if the need arises, identify who the relevant information should be shared with to prevent potential self-harm by the participant. Furthermore, a management plan and safeguarding mechanisms for the potential harms to others or the risk of breaching prison security need to be developed with the same considerations.

However, the overtly risk-adverse approach to research within prisons has been questioned. In the UK, current guidance has been described as 'protectionist' and prisoners are rarely offered access to participate in research, and perhaps this will now be challenged to allow prisoners access to research in line with the ethical principle of equivalence in prison health and social care (Charles et al., 2016).

9.2 PATIENT AND PUBLIC INVOLVEMENT

Patient and public involvement (PPI) supports the development of research 'with' or even 'by' members of the public, rather than research being 'done to' or 'about' or 'for them' (Bagley et al., 2016). PPI supports people who are being researched to have a voice and influence the decisions regarding the development of research. This is important as the implementation of the recommendations from research may directly affect their support or care. A slogan, which is thought to be over five centuries old, has been adopted by Dementia Alliance International (DAI) within research and any decisions made about people with dementia is 'nothing about us without us' (DAI, 2015). The concept of PPI addresses a number of ethical issues including respect for autonomy, beneficence and non-maleficence. The respect for autonomy is addressed through the engagement of members of the population being researched. Within the prison setting, this may include prisoners, and their involvement would support the development of research they would find acceptable to participate in, and findings and possible recommendations relevant to their needs. The application of PPI also supports the two principles of risk analysis, beneficence and non-maleficence, as within prison research, prisoners and other stakeholders will be able to become involved in the risk analysis and discuss their understanding and views, which may be from different perspectives.

10 Dissemination policy

The dissemination policy is an important part of the protocol, as it identifies who owns the data or intellectual property, which arises from the research when the study has been completed. On completion of the research, a Final Study Report should be disseminated with the relevant research committees and other regulatory bodies who provided approval, including the governor of the prison where data collection occurred. Finally, how the outcomes and recommendations of the study are going to be provided to all those who participated in the research needs to be identified. This may be the Final Study Report, publications or a specifically designed newsletter or presentation.

Ethics in practice in prison research

Guidelines to support research in prison settings and with prisoners have been published. Innes (2003) suggest six practical steps are necessary before starting a research project; each of these will be discussed in depth and developed further to explore and highlight ethical issues that may arise during research with prisoners in the prison setting:

Stakeholder engagement

Stakeholder holder engagement was briefly discussed in the previous section under PPI as well as the importance of obtaining stakeholder engagement to shape the research proposal to meet the overarching needs of the prison. Stakeholders within prison researcher have been defined as 'individuals who have a stake in the prison population, the capacity to affect and facilitate change at a systems level' (Wakai et al., 2009). This definition of stakeholders identifies two important aspects, the ability to support research access and implement the recommendations of change from the research. Therefore, it is essential to obtain stakeholder engagement during the development of the research, which includes the governor of a prison, who can ultimately restrict access. An approach to obtain and maintain stakeholder engagement is through inviting them to join a steering group for the duration of the research. A steering group involves experts within research to ensure the protocol is followed but also involves PPI engagement, including members from the population being stud-ied and relevant stakeholders. A steering group will meet at a number of key stages during the implementation of the research and can influence strategic decisions, therefore maintaining stakeholder engagement, which is not overly burdensome for the stakeholders.

However, prison officers are ultimately the 'gate keepers' to prisoners, and approval for research by prison administration might not translate into either their cooperation or support to access to areas of the prison or prisoners. Prison officers can block access to prisoners for a variety of reasons and in a variety of ways (Waldram, 1998). Often the relationship between prison officers and researchers is uneasy one (Sparks et al., 1996). The perspective of the prison officers needs to be considered. They are responsible for the order of the prison, which can be a dangerous environment, and the implementation of research within this environment may cause disruption to the safety and well-being of prisoners and prison officers (Roberts and Indermaur, 2008).

Prison officers as gatekeepers may select prisoners to participate in research, who may significantly differ from other prisoners in a number of ways. Selected prisoners may advocate an agenda prisoner officers are interested in raising at a higher level, or prisoners may be volunteering to gain favour with the prison officers. Prison officers may inadvertently bias the research by influenc-ing the recruitment process through passing negative comments to researchers regarding individual prisoners (Waldram, 1998). Additionally, if prison officers express negative comments regarding the research to prisoners and that they or the prison governor are not in favour of the research, this is likely to deter pris-oners from participating. Therefore, there are a number of elements that can lead to recruitment bias if prison officers are directly involved, which needs to be considered when developing both sampling and recruitment of participants (Roberts and Indermaur, 2008).

Inclusion of an experienced prison researcher

A further practical step in the development of prison research is the need to have at least one researcher who is experienced in the completion of research in a prison setting. This approach will provide confidence to ethical, regulatory bodies and prison boards that the research team will have an understanding of the prison culture and how to implement research in prison setting success-fully (Apa et al., 2012). The inclusion of an experienced prison researcher can support and mentor more junior members of the team, especially when they are working through different emotions and feelings of safety and their own well-being, alongside how to react to, and when or if information regarding criminal activity needs to be disclosed (Lucic-Catic, 2011).

University or institution support

Researchers need to obtain assistance from their university or institution. This is important for two reasons. First, the researcher's own institution needs to provide approval for the study to be conducted by a member of their staff, as their responsibility is to be the sponsor of the study, and provide indemnity, which is the insurance to cover a possible complaint or harm as a result of the research. Second, the researcher's institution can provide assistance with the completion of documentation to obtain external ethical approval and prison approval from the relevant institutions.

Research to address the mission statement of the prison

The research must address the mission statement of the prison and consider relevant prison policies and the current issues identified both nationally and regionally. The understanding of the mission statement and the current needs of prisons can be further understood by engaging with administration staff, healthcare professionals, prison staff and officers and prisoners where possible. This approach will support the development of research with mutual goals and commence the collaborative relationship between researchers and those working in the prison (Apa et al., 2012). An important consideration, which has been acknowledged previously, is the need to engage with prison officers and understand how the research will disrupt the everyday operations of the prison, especially the need to move individual prisoners around the prison. The involvement of prison officers in the design of the study and allowing them to influence some of the decisions being made, such as when and where interviews or focus groups may occur, are likely to support the smooth running of the research (Apa et al., 2012)

Understanding the ethical approval process

It is important to understand the ethical approval process – and the extra layers of formal and informal processes in gaining access to conduct healthcare research in prison with prisoners – and the delays that may occur at any step of the process.

Commence with a pilot study

An ideal way of demonstrating the value of research is to commence with a pilot study, which will also support the development and feasibility of the research. There are four main aspects of a pilot study to support that address the feasibility of conducting a full study: recruitment, testing the questionnaires or measurement, and data entry and analysis (Hassan et al., 2006). Recruitment has to some extent been addressed previously. However, it is also important to understand if potential participants would be interested in participating in this research. Another important element is understanding the relevance of the questionnaires or measurements to the study population, especially when these are self-completed by participants. A pilot study will identify if the questionnaires or questions within an interview or focus group are clearly understood by potential participants. A pilot study will also identify if the information provided in the participant information sheet contains an appropriate level of language without any complex medical terms that potential participants can understand. Issues raised during the pilot study may include the identification of questions that have an ambiguous meaning or poorly understood by potential participants, questions that were not in a logical order, too many questions causing the potential participants to lose interest and questions that either the potential participants did not want to answer or were unexpectedly sensitive in nature. From these observations and other comments by potential participants, the questionnaire or question route for interviews and focus groups can be amended to be more appropriate and engaging for future participants. The completion of a pilot study will inform and amend the protocol and ensure the successful completion of the full study.

Summary

This chapter has discussed the four pillars of biomedical ethics with relevance to research in the prison population. It highlighted some of the complexities of applying ethical research in a closed and coercive environment. It also discussed the need for prisoners not to be 'overprotected' and to be provided the opportunity to participate in research as they would if they were living in the community. Research exploring health and social care provision with prisons is essential to support health and social care professionals in delivering evidence-based care. The final elements of this chapter have provided guidance on who to write an ethical protocol for a qualitative study recruiting participants within a prison setting, with reference to and consideration of the four pillars of biomedical ethics. Lastly, this chapter has provided some practical advice on enabling the successful completion of the research.

References

Abbott, L., Scott, T. (2018). Reflections in researcher departure: closure of prison relationships in ethnographic research. *Nursing Ethics*, 26(5): 1424–1441.

Ahalt, C., Sudore, R., Bolano, M., Metzger, L., Darby, A.M., Williams, B. (2017). "Teach-to-goal" to better assess informed consent comprehension among incarcerated clinical research participants. *AMA Journal of Ethics*, 19(9): 862–872.

Andorno, R., Shaw, D.M., Elger, B. (2015). Protecting prisoners' autonomy with advance directives. Ethical dilemmas and policy issues. *Medicine, Health Care and Philosophy*, 18: 33–39.

Apa, Z.L., Bai, R.Y., Mukherejee, D.V., Herzig, C.T.A., Koenigsmann, C., Lowy, F.D., Larson, E.L. (2012). Challenges and strategies for research in Prisons. *Public Health Nursing*, 29(5): 467–472.

Applebaum, K.L., Hickey, J.M., Packer, I. (2001). The role of correctional officers in multi-disciplinary mental health care in prisons. *Psychiatric Services*, 52: 1343–1347.

Bagley, H.J., Short, H., Harman, N.L., Hickey, H.R., Gamble, C.L., Woolfall, K., Young, B., Williamson, P.R. (2016). A patient and public involvement (PPI) toolkit for meaningful and flexible involvement in clinical trials – a work in progress. *Research Involvement and Engagement*, 2: 15.

Beauchamp, T.L., Childress, J.F. (2001). *Principles of Biomedical Ethics*. 5th edition. Oxford: Oxford University Press.

Belmont Report (1979). Ethical principles and guidelines for the protection of human subjects of research. Available from: www.hhs.gov/ohrp/regulations-and-policy/belmont-report/index.html [Assessed on: 24 May 2020].

Binswanger, I.A., Krueger, P.M., Steiner, J.F. (2009). Prevalence of chronic medical conditions among jail and prison inmates in the USA compared with the general population. *Journal of Epidemiology and Community Health*, 63(11): 912–919.

Braun, V., Clarke, V. (2006). Using thematic analysis in psychology. *Qualitative Research in Psychology*, 3(2): 77–101.

Brooke, J., Rybacka, M. (2020). Development of a dementia education workshop for prison staff, prisoners, and health and social care professionals to enable them to support prisoners with dementia. *Journal of Correctional Health Care*, DOI: 10.1177/1078345820916444.

Charles, A., Rid, A., Davies, H., Draper, H. (2016). Prisoners as research participants: current practice and attitudes in the UK. *Journal of Medical Ethics*, 42: 246–252.

Coninx, R., Maher, D., Reyes, H., Grzemska, M. (2000). Tuberculosis in prisons in countries with high prevalence. *BMJ*, 320(7232): 440–442.

Copes, H., Hochstetler, A., Brown, A. (2012). Inmates' perceptions of the benefits and harm of prison interviews. *Field Matters*, 25: 182–196.

Council of Europe (2005). *Additional Protocol to the Convention on Human Rights and Biomedicine, Concerning Biomedical Research*. Available from: www.coe.int/en/web/bioethics/biomedical-research [Accessed on: 24 May 2020].

Cowburn, M. (2005). Confidentiality and public protection: ethical dilemmas in qualitative research with adult male sex offenders. *Journal of Sexual Aggression*, 11(1): 49–63.

Daley, K. (2015). The wrongs of prosecution: balancing protection and participation in research with marginalised young people. *Journal of Sociology*, 51: 121–138.

de Montmollin, M.J. (1985). Treatment of personality disorders? The sociotherapy workshop of the medical department of Clamp-Dollon prison (Geneva): 5-year survey. *Revue Medicale Suisse*, 105(1): 65–71.

Dementia Alliance International (2015). *Nothing About Us Without Us*. Available from: www.dementiaallianceinternational.org/nothing-about-us-without-us/ [Accessed on: 24 May 2020].

Dworkin, S.L. (2012). Sample size policy for quantitative studies using in-depth interviews. *Archives of Sexual Behaviour*, 41: 1319–1320.

Gale, N.K., Heath, G., Cameron, E., Rashid, S., Redwood, S. (2013). Using the framework method for the analysis of qualitative data in multi-disciplinary health research. *BMC Medical Research Methodology*, 13: 117.

Giordano, J., O'Reilly, M., Taylor, H., Dogra, N. (2007). Confidentiality and Autonomy: the challenge(s) of offering research participants a choice of disclosing their identity. *Qualitative Health Research*, 17(2): 264–275.

Glaser, B.G., Strauss, A.L. (1967). *The Discovery of Grounded Theory: Strategies for Qualitative Research*. Chicago: Aldine Publishing Co.

Hassan, Z., Schattner, P., Mazza, D. (2006). Doing a pilot study: why is it essential? *Malaysian Family Physician*, 1(2–3): 70–73.

Herbert, K., Plugge, E., Foster, C., Doll, H. (2012). Prevalence of risk factors for non-communicable diseases in prison populations worldwide: a systematic review. *The Lancet*, 1975–1982.

Innes, C.A. (2003). *Learning Lessons and Lessons Learned: The National Institute of Justice's Research Demonstration Project Strategy*. Paper prepared for the annual meetings of the Academy of Criminal Justice Sciences, Boston.

Kazdin, A.E. (1977). Assessing the clinical or applied importance of behaviour change through social validation. *Behaviour Modification*, 1: 427–452.

King, H., Measham, F., O'Brien, K. (2019). Building bridges across diversity: utilising the inside-out prison exchange programme to promote an egalitarian higher education community within three English prisons. *The International Journal of Bias, Identity and Diversities in Education*, 4(1): 66–81.

Labott, S.M., Johnson, T.P., Fendrich, M., Feeny, N. (2013). Emotional risks to respondents in survey research: some empirical evidence. *Journal of Empirical Research on Human Research Ethics*, 8(4): 53–66.

Lahm, K.F. (2009). Inmate assaults on prison staff: a multilevel examination of an overlooked form of prison violence. *The Prison Journal*, 89(2): 131–150.

Lammy Review (2017). *An Independent Review into the Treatment of, and Outcomes for, Black, Asian and Minority Ethnic Individuals in the Criminal Justice System*. Available from: https://assets.publishing.service.gov.uk/government/uploads/system/uploads/attachment_data/file/643001/lammy-review-final-report.pdf [Accessed on: 24 May 2020].

Liabo, K., Ingold, A., Roberts, H. (2017). Co-production with "vulnerable" groups: balancing protection and participation. *Health Science Reports*, e19.

Lucic-Catic, M. (2011). Challenges in conducting prison research. *Journal of Criminal Justice and Security*, XI(5–6): 59–73.

Macklin, R. (2014). Ethical challenges in implementation research. *Public Health Ethics*, 7(1): 86–93.

Martin, R.E., Chan, R., Torrika, L., Grange-Brown, A., Ramsden, V.R. (2008). Healing fostered by research. *Canadian Family Physician*, 54: 244–245.

Mason, M. (2010). Sample size and saturation in PhD studies using qualitative interviews. *Forum: Qualitative Social Research*, 11(3): 8.

Ralphs, R., Williams, L., Askewa, R., Norton, A. (2017). Adding spice to the porridge: the development of a synthetic cannabinoid market in an English prison. *International Journal of Drug Policy*, 40: 57–69.

Roberts, L., Indermaur, D. (2008). The ethics of research with prisoners. *Current Issues in Criminal Justice*, 19(3): 309–326.

Ryan, R.M., Deci, E.L. (2000). Self-determination theory and the facilitation of intrinsic motivation, social development and well-being. *American Psychologist*, 55: 68–78.

Schlosser, J.A. (2008). Issues in interviewing inmates. *Qualitative Inquiry*, 14(8): 1300–1525.

Shaw, D., Elger, B. (2015). Improving health by respecting autonomy: using social science research to enfranchise vulnerable prison populations. *Preventative Medicine*, 74: 21–23.

Smith, J.A., Flowers, P., Larkin, M. (2009). *Interpretative Phenomenological Analysis: Theory, Method and Research*. London: Sage Publications.

Smoyer, A.B. (2019). Teaching note – taking social work undergraduates inside: the Inside-Out Prison Exchange Program. *Journal of Social Work Education*, 56(1): 186–192.

Sparks, R., Bottoms, A.E., Hay, W. (1996). *Prisons and the Problems of Order*. Oxford: Clarendon Press.

Spencer, S.-J. (2017). Striving for balance between participation and protection in research involving prison populations. *Australian and New Zealand Journal of Psychiatry*, 51(10): 974–976.

Thomson, N.D., Vassileva, J., Kiehl, K.A., Reidy, D., Aboutanosa, M., McDouglee, R., DeLisi, M. (2019). Which features of psychopathy and impulsivity matter most for prison violence? New evidence among female prisoners. *International Journal of Law and Psychiatry*, 64: 29–33.

Thrasher, J., Maloney, E., Mills, S., House, J., Wroe, T., White, V. (2019). Reimaging prison research from inside-out. *Journal of Prisoners on Prisons*, 28(1): 12–27.

van der Kaap-Deeder, J., Audenaert, E., van Mastrigt, S., Mabbe, E., Vansteenkiste, M. (2017). Choosing when choices are limited: the role of perceived afforded choice and autonomy in prisoners' well-being. *Law and Human Behavior*, 41(6): 567–578.

Wakai, S., Shelton, D., Trestman, R.L., Kesten, K. (2009). Conducting research in corrections: challenges and solutions. *Behaviour Sciences and Law*, 27: 743–752.

Waldram, J. (1998). Anthropology in prison: negotiating consent and accountability with a "captured" population. *Human Organization*, 57(2): 238–244.

Ward, J., Bailey, D. (2012). Consent, confidentiality and ethics in PAR in the context of prison research. *Ethics in Social Research*, 12: 149–169.

Weild, A.R., Gill, O.N., Bennett, D., Livingstone, S.J.M., Parry, J.V., Curran, L. (2000). Prevalence of HIV, hepatitis B, and hepatitis C antibodies in prisoners in England and Wales: a national survey. *Communicable Diseases Public Health*, 3(2): 121–126.

Wester, K.L. (2011). Publishing ethical research: a step-by-step overview. *Journal of Counselling and Development*, 89: 301–307.

Wolf, M.M. (1978). Social validity: the case for subjective measurement or how applied behaviour analysis is finding its heart. *Journal of Applied Behaviour Analysis*, 11: 203–214.

World Medical Association (1964). *WMA Declaration of Helsinki – Ethical Principles of Medical Research Involving Human Subjects*. Available from: www.wma.net/wp-content/uploads/2018/07/DoH-Jun1964.pdf [Accessed on: 24 May 2020].

9 Recommendations

Joanne Brooke

Healthcare provision for older prisoners and those with dementia

This section will include an overview of current issues as highlighted in the relevant chapters, followed by a discussion and recommendations to support and address all issues raised.

Aging prison population

Many countries across the world are seeing an increase in the average age of those in prison, with older prisoners the fastest-growing group within prison populations. Figures regarding prisoners over the age of 50 in prisons in England and Wales, the USA and Australia were presented in Chapter 1. In the Prison Service of England and Wales, prisoners over the age of 50 are predicted to increase in both absolute terms and as a proportion of the overall prison population. This is partly because of the worldwide aging population. In countries such as the UK, the USA and Australia, the dominant method of punishment for crime is imprisonment, although this is only one reason why prison populations are aging. Further reasons in England and Wales include custodial sentences for breaches of bail, and long prison terms, those over 10 years. Because of the convictions of historical sex crimes, prisoners are now entering prison when they are 70 years old and over.

The definition of an older prisoner has only just begun to be discussed; it needs to be evidence-based and represent the negative impact of prison on prisoner's physical and mental well-being as well as their health and social care needs, as the definition informs both policy and practice. In the Prison Service of England and Wales, the accepted definition is now any prisoner over the age of 50. This is because of the accelerated aging of prisoners, with prison having a negative impact on their physical and mental health. Other factors that affect the health of older prisoners include poor health and lifestyle choices before and during a prison sentence, significant trauma, grief and loss, social disadvantage and lower levels of education. There is a need to recognise that the health and social care needs of prisoners should be considered complex from a younger age, as their functionality may not correspond with their chronological age. Therefore, the provision of health and social care services are required to address a number of emerging issues regarding older prisoners and their poor health, which were previously not prevalent, and one of these is dementia.

In the Prison Service of England and Wales, it has been recognised and acknowledged, that at the time of writing, there remains the need for the development and implementation of a national strategy for older prisoners. A number of independent organisations have called for a strategy to encompass older prisoners and those with disabilities including cognitive impairment, to support the formulation of a clear pathway for all prisons, their governors and healthcare providers to implement, alongside clear and identifiable standards that need to be met. The identification of older prisoners and their health and social needs, which are unique and complex compared to their younger counterparts, has been the focus of discussion in England and Wales for over a decade. Therefore, there is now a clear need and rationale for a national strategy to support older prisoners. This is a recommendation that has been widely acknowledged.

One call for a national strategy for older prisoners was by the Prison Reform Trust (2019), which suggests that the HM Prison and Probation Service is responsible for such development, and provides in-depth information on the recommended content of the strategy. Recommendations include the need for a complete descriptive profile of older people in prison; the development for standards of care for older people in custody, including the need for practical implications of their legal status; guidance on purposeful activities for older prison, encompassing work, leisure and activities, providing older people with the same, but appropriate opportunities as younger prisoners; the need for education and training of all personnel who come into contact with older prisoners, including legal, prison and health and social care staff; the development of information-sharing protocols, especially between healthcare professionals and prison staff; the recognition and provision of services that are required by older prisoners, such as physiotherapy and occupation therapy to support mobility and the provision of aids to promote independence; and an element that was discussed in some depth within the provision of healthcare in prison is the acknowledgement of the challenges of providing palliative and end-of-life care within a prison, and determining whether a prison is the most suitable environment when end-of-life care is required.

An essential recommendation is the development of mandated requirements for prisons that will hold people over the age of 50, and the responsibilities of all agencies to ensure age-appropriate treatment and services are provided during custody and continued upon their release. Within this recommendation, it is essential that, as per prison healthcare guidelines, healthcare professionals actively seek to identify any health conditions, which needs to include dementia. Older prisoners who have developed cognitive impairment during their prison stay and are released without this impairment acknowledged will not have a successful resettlement and the care and support they require will not have been put in place. Because of the nature of the crimes of some older prisoners who have entered prison for the first time in their later years, there is probably no family or friends to support them on their release, and it is likely that a condition of their release is that they are not permitted to return to their home town. Therefore, a number of older prisoners may be released to an unfamiliar town with no support from family or friends, and no support from health and social care professionals as their cognitive impairment was not recognised before their release. This needs to be addressed urgently through national and local strategies, protocols and pathways.

Healthcare provision in prison

The World Health Organization in 2014 highlighted 12 essential principles of healthcare in prison settings, which recognise both the human rights of prisoners and the provision of ethical healthcare. These have been discussed in Chapter 2. In Europe, the roles of healthcare professionals in the provision of healthcare in prison settings has been explicitly stated. Healthcare professionals are responsible for the diagnosis of both physical and mental health conditions, for the provision of treatment for prisoners whilst in prison and for identifying physical or psychological limitations that may affect a prisoner's resettlement following release. These responsibilities need to include the identification and diagnosis of dementia. In the Prison Service of England and Wales, healthcare provision is the responsibility of five partners: the Ministry of Justice, Her Majesty's Prison and Probation Service, Public Health England, the Department of Health and Social Care and NHS England. These institutions have outlined clear aims and objectives for improving the provision of healthcare in prison, and the commissioning of healthcare services removed from prison administrations to NHS Foundation Trusts. However, prisoners are still not obtaining healthcare provision that is equitable to the general population.

Access to healthcare by prisoners is an ongoing concern, and in Chapter 2 it was highlighted that 40 per cent of outpatient appointments for prisoners went unattended. There are many reasons for this, some of which are unavoidable and some related to limited resources, so new ways of delivering external healthcare to prisoners is urgently required to support both prisoners' health and aid the efficiency of the NHS. Healthcare provision within the community is changing to incorporate new ways of working with the advancement of technology, which support both efficiency and the ability of those who are unable to commute to the primary or secondary healthcare setting. One development is the use of video conferencing, and 3 per cent of outpatient appointments were completed through this approach. This approach could be further developed to support prisoners to attend hospital appointments 'virtually' as this would remove the need for two prison officers to escort the prison to physically attend the appointment and could occur in the presence of a healthcare professional to support the continuity of care. In a recent study, only 2 per cent of outpatient appointments with prisoners occurred 'virtually', which is less than those completed by people living in the community. This needs to be addressed urgently to enable prisoners to access healthcare.

Challenges remain in the provision of healthcare in the prison setting, including the provision of chronic disease management, because of the need for specialist care for a number of diseases, which has not been possible due to a lack of resources to employ or access in-reach services that provide such specialist care. Currently, healthcare professionals especially nurses, who lead clinics, are specialised in one chronic disease, and have general knowledge regarding other chronic diseases. This approach needs to be addressed to support nurses in acquiring in-depth knowledge of a number of chronic diseases. It is recognised, however, that this approach is not supported in non-correctional healthcare provision. Nurses have also identified the conflict between opposing cultures of custody and care, and the need to negotiate boundaries between these two cultures, which affected the care they provided. Other challenges identified have included the need to create a caring environment in the prison setting, the need to remain vigilant around convicted offenders and the attitude and language of correction staff, but overwhelmingly nurses discussed the uncomfortable feeling they experienced when the security of the prison was prioritised over the care they needed to provide to a patient. This element has begun to be addressed through education and training of both prison staff and nurses to support an understanding of each other's roles, and prison officers dedicated to work within the healthcare facilities within a prison.

Dementia

An overview of dementia has been provided in Chapter 3, with the introduction of Alzheimer's disease, vascular dementia, dementia with Lewy bodies, Alcohol Related Brain Damage and Wernicke-Korsakoff syndrome. All of these types of dementia have different presentations and require a different formal diagnosis from specialists in the field of dementia, such as old age psychiatrist, to support the treatment for the explicit type of dementia identified. An overview of the different symptoms of each of these main types of dementia was also presented. However, the important element for healthcare professionals and prison staff is the ability to understand the different early symptoms of dementia and to enable appropriate screening and referral for a full cognitive assessment (this process will be further addressed in the next section). Healthcare professionals and prison staff need to be aware of the pharmacological treatment for dementia and that drugs are available to slow the progression of the disease, and thereby support the person with dementia to live independently and without care for longer. This is important to address within prison settings as prison staff have identified they lack knowledge regarding dementia, and with this the misconception that there is no treatment for dementia, although it must be recognised that there is no cure.

The principles of person-centred care have been introduced in Chapter 2 and include giving a person with dementia dignity, respect and compassion;

providing coordinated care, support and treatment; providing personalised care, support and treatment; and enabling a person. These principles have been recognised in the care of the person with dementia since 2015. However, they have yet to be fully embedded in all health and social care provisions, including hospitals, primary care and resident/nursing homes, as well as places of detention. The provision of person-centred care is a philosophy of care built around the needs of the person with dementia and is contingent on knowing the person through an interpersonal relationship and respecting an individual's personhood. In the community, this process is supported with the involvement of family members and close friends. However, in the prison environment, family members and close friends may need to be temporarily replaced by fellow prisoners, as neither prison staff nor healthcare professionals will have the time or capacity to build this relationship, and family members and friends will not have enough visitation rights to continue this relationship. This is discussed further in the next section.

An element that is important to both appreciate and understand within dementia is that once you have met one person with dementia, you still only have met one person with dementia. This is because dementia is a disease that affects each individually differently, and the journey for each individual will be different. This is important because care and interventions to support someone to live well with dementia need to be personalised or individualised for that person and are not appropriate to all people with dementia. All human beings are individuals and have different preferences, and this needs to be considered when planning to support and care for a person with dementia. Person-centred models of care need to include the value of a person with dementia, to respect them and those who care for them, treating the person with dementia as an individual, to see the world from the perspective of the person with dementia, and to provide a positive social environment in which the person with dementia can experience relative well-being. The concepts need to be applied in all environments that support people with dementia, and this includes the prison setting. Initiatives have begun to address these issues which have been described in Chapter 4.

Lastly, there is a need to understand changes in behaviour in people with dementia, and this is the most complex aspect of supporting such persons. Behaviours can be exacerbated when a person with dementia is feeling confused or distressed and trying to make sense of what is happening, or when they are trying to communicate their needs. Within the confined constraints of a prison setting, changes in behaviour that may challenge the prison regime may occur because of a prisoner's dementia, and this needs to be recognised and responded to appropriately. One approach that supports behaviours of people with dementia is the adoption of a formulation-led model, such as the Newcastle Clinical Model, which includes a range of information to consider, such as physical and mental health, the environment, as well as the life story and personality of the person, to assist in the understanding of thoughts, emotions and beliefs underlying the person's change in behaviour. The Newcastle Clinical

Model is appropriate for all environments and can be implemented within the prison environment with the support of other prisoners, prison officers and health and social care professionals.

Initiatives to support prisoners with dementia

This element will provide an overview of the current initiatives that were explored in earlier chapters that aim to support older prisoners and those with dementia. This will also include a discussion on the practical implications of these initiatives, which will be informed by the author's own experience. However, it will be highlighted that further implementation of similar initiatives needs to occur alongside a robust evaluation, which includes the impact on the prisoner, the prison regime, sustainability and cost-effectiveness.

An overview of dementia in prison settings has been provided in Chapter 4, and the estimated prevalence of dementia in prison settings, alongside the prisoners' increased risk factors of developing dementia. Currently, there appears to be a discrepancy between the risk factors, poor health of prisoners and the prevalence of dementia within prison settings. A number of reasons may be responsible for this discrepancy, including the lack of a sensitive cognitive screening tool to specifically identify dementia in those who are serving in a prison setting. There is a need for the development of a cognitive screening tool appropriate to prison environments in England and Wales, one has been developed in the US, but this is not transferable, as the prison regimes are significantly different. An appropriate cognitive screening tool, which is sensitive to and identifies subtle changes in prisoner's cognitive abilities will support the identification of prisoners who require further cognitive assessment. Alongside the development of a cognitive screening tool explicitly for the prison setting is the need for cognitive screening to occur more frequently than just on admission to a prison, or if an issue has been identified. In line with equitable healthcare in the community, prisoners over the age of 50, rather than 65 as in the community, should be offered cognitive screening every 12 months throughout their prison sentence. This process will support the early identification in cognitive changes in prisoners.

The importance of early identification of cognitive changes in prisoners can only be partially reinforced by an appropriate cognitive screening, which needs to be supported through a clear and transparent pathway. On completion of an appropriate cognitive screening tool and an identification of a possible change in cognitive abilities, there needs to be an identified pathway to refer the prisoner for further cognitive assessment, whether this provision is provided within the prison or externally. Within prisons in England and Wales, the first point of referral if the cognitive screen was completed by a nurse would be to arrange an appointment with a GP responsible for the prisoner. This would support the investigation of other physical or psychological causes of the identified cognitive changes, and the GP would complete a medical history with the prisoner and a series of blood tests as per national guidelines. Once the information and test results are obtained, the prisoner will be referred to a consultant psychiatrist; within prisons in England and Wales, this would occur within the prison setting.

Initiatives within prison settings to support prisoners with dementia have begun to be developed and a number of these initiatives from around the world that are considered 'gold standard' have been described in Chapter 4. Models of delivering social care in prison have also begun to be formulated and described (Maschi et al., 2012; Lee et al., 2016, 2019). From these models and the need to support prisoners with dementia, four main components have been identified that should to be considered in the development of initiatives: environment, education, meaningful engagement and collaboration and support. Each of these will now be considered in more depth alongside recommendations.

Environment

Prison environments, especially in England and Wales, have been discussed in a number of chapters. The unsuitable environments of prisons built in the Victoria era continue to affect all prisoners held in these prisons. However, for a prisoner with dementia, added difficulties are experienced, as these prisons can be noisy and overwhelming. A prison initiative for prisoners with dementia needs to address the environment, with the consideration of the following, although it is recognised some of these will be difficult to implement:

- Accessibility is an important factor to maintain a prisoner's independence and may include the need to provide handrails, doors accessible by wheelchairs, specialities facilities for showering and dining, all being on the same level.
- Signposting provide clear direction for the prisoner with dementia and may alleviate potential confusion and again support their independence. Signposting and labelling need to include large print and pictures, arrows along the floor to direct a prisoner to the toilet, possibly individualisation such as a photograph of the prison and their name on their cell door.
- Sensory environment needs to be considered as it can be overwhelming for prisoners with dementia, with harsh lighting and loud noises, which could trigger behaviour that would challenge the prison regime. Adaptations could include bright but not harsh lighting, and a quiet space for prisoners who are showing signs of being overwhelmed.
- Personal care may need to be supported through the provision of clothing that is easy to put on and off, signage and pictures for activities to highlight routines and the allocation of a peer for further guidance and support.

Education

As previously mentioned in Chapter 4, there is a need for training and education of prison staff, prisoners and healthcare professionals to recognise symptoms of dementia within a prison regime. Therefore, any initiative to support prisoners with dementia must have an element of training and education, not only those involved in the initiative, but more widely across the prison, to support a prison-wide understanding. Elements of training and education must encompass dementia awareness, recognising signs and symptoms and managing behaviour and effective communication, with the consideration of the following:

- Dementia awareness is an essential component for all staff and prisoners, including governors, as it can improve their knowledge of this syndrome, alongside dispelling some negative myths.
- Recognising signs and symptoms is essential for an early and prompt referral; training and education should not only include the signs and symptoms of dementia, but the referral process when concerns are identified.
- Managing behaviour which can be challenging for the person with dementia, staff and the prison regime, clear advice and support are required on how to identify triggers for individual prisoners with dementia and the development of care plans that will support staff to support the prisoner with dementia.
- Effective communication is essential in supporting prisoners with dementia; therefore, the provision of a range of tools to support communication, including non-verbal materials need to be explained and provided.

Meaningful engagement

Meaningful engagement or purposeful activity is the engagement of a prisoner with dementia and not a tokenistic approach of keeping the person with dementia busy. Activities can support and promote independence, through both physical and mental exercises created specifically for prisoners with dementia. The development of meaningful engagement or purposeful activity for prisoners with dementia should consider the following:

- Support from other prisoners, who can provide meaningful engagement for a prisoner with dementia, whilst developing their role as social care providers.
- Physical activities that are age appropriate can be adapted for prisoners with dementia, which will improve health and mental well-being.
- Social engagement can be incorporated in a variety of ways, including the provision of activities such as pet therapy, singing and reminiscence.
- Activities that support cognitive functioning are important to both defer further cognitive decline and maintain meaningful engagement; these activities need to stimulate cognitive process, such as art, music and discussions at a level appropriate for each prisoner with dementia.
- Communication encourages engagement and should be casual to encourage the prisoner to engage, which will support relationships between prisoners with dementia and their peer support and prison staff.

Collaboration and support

The implementation of initiatives to support prisoners with dementia requires collaboration and support from both prison staff and prisoners as well as outside agencies, such as social care and physiotherapy and occupational therapy. Currently lacking in the development of a number of initiatives to support prisoners with dementia is the inclusion of an occupational therapist who can provide support and advice in the majority of areas necessary to assist a person with dementia and involve them in meaningful engagement and purposeful activities. A collaborative approach for the development of initiatives to support prisoners with dementia needs to consider and identify a core team of staff and prisoners, healthcare professionals, social services and external agencies, which are now discussed in more detail:

- Core team of staff and prisoners will provide contact points for support and information; the value of having fellow prisoners to support prisoners with dementia has been identified in a number of initiatives and has been described as buddying.
- Healthcare professionals' involvement is essential and should involve a range of professionals whose expertise is in the field of dementia to support both prisoners with dementia, fellow prisoners and staff with any concerns or issues raised.
- Social services also have a vast experience of assessing the needs of individuals with dementia and should be included in any initiative, although this is currently not routine practice in prisons in England and Wales.
- External agencies such as Alzheimer's Society, Dementia UK and Age UK all offer support to prisoners with dementia, and it is important to engage with these charities to enable them to provide regular and consistent support. In a number of prisons in the UK, Alzheimer's Society has supported the delivery of dementia friends' sessions to raise the awareness of dementia in the prison setting. For prisons with financial restraints, the engagement with charitable agencies is an essential approach to support initiatives for prisoner with dementia

Finally, there is a need to develop this suggested framework, not only to support the development and implementation of prison initiatives to support prisoners with dementia, but also to provide a robust evaluation of these initiatives, which is lacking. Currently, there is no data to understand the impact of these initiatives on the prisoner with dementia, prison and healthcare staff, other prisoners and the prison regime. The current support for these initiatives is all anecdotal. Furthermore, anecdotal information does not provide an understanding of the financial benefits, sustainability or the long-term impact of these initiatives. Therefore, an essential recommendation is further research in this area to identify the measurable outcomes and impacts of these initiatives.

Robust ethical research on dementia in prison

The first part of this element will draw on the chapters that have highlighted the need for further research in the prison setting to understand the impact of dementia, highlighting the urgent need for current robust research to address the numerous questions that remain unanswered. The second part of this element will draw conclusions from the chapters addressing research ethics in a prison setting. Recommendations and guidance on research processes including ethics will provide potential researchers on dementia in the prison setting an insight into researching a subject (dementia) that remains misunderstood and underrepresented in research, with the added complication of completing the research in a prison setting.

Healthcare provisions in prison settings have improved significantly over the last decade, but there remains a need for evidence-based healthcare to be implemented. Therefore, clinical research, including health and social care research, needs to support the development of an evidence base for healthcare provision relevant to the prison setting. However, because of the historical contexts of prison research, there are unique challenges to this approach, as structure, ethical principles and access to prisoners have become restricted, leaving prisoners overprotected and understudied. The ethical principles and those developed specifically for the inclusion of prisoners in research are essential to protect prisoners from exploitation. However, within the prison setting and including prisoners in research, there is still a need for a clear understanding of exploitation, as prison environments do not naturally support prisoners to make autonomous decisions.

An important issue is that of obtaining informed consent, and there remains a need to develop a process of obtaining consent which focuses on the protection of prisoners from coercion, independence of the researchers from routine healthcare professionals or prison administration, with a clear and detailed provision of the limits and risks as well of benefits of participating in research. The challenges of obtaining informed consent have been discussed in Chapter 7. The development of a formal process still needs to occur, which considers the elements of autonomy, including confidentiality and autonomy, protection and autonomy and perceived afforded choice and autonomy with an environment which is inherently coercive, which have been discussed in Chapter 8.

The development of an ethical protocol for research in the prison setting has also been discussed in detail in Chapter 8, and it is recommended that any research within a prison setting needs to incorporate these ethical considerations, which are summarised in the following table. Table 9.1 is a summary of the information to support the development of an ethical protocol for prison research and how the four ethical principles can be both identified and addressed within elements of the protocol. Some mandatory elements of a protocol have not been included as they are factual elements that need to be completed for all research and are not specific for the development of research in a prison setting.

Table 9.1 An overview of developing a qualitative ethical protocol for prison research

Component of protocol	Ethical principle	Application
Rationale	Justice	Justification and social validity of the study are required to meet the needs and aims of prisoners and the prison, to support equity and equality of access and provision of health and social care
Theoretical Framework	Beneficence	The reliability and validity of research is supported through the application of a theoretical framework, which supports the ethical and informed approach of data collection, analysis and recommendations
Aims, objectives and outcomes	Autonomy	These do not incidentally explore information that may include unprosecuted criminal activity or activity that might affect the security of the prison
Study design	Beneficence	The design must identify which of the four qualitative research designs, phenomenology, ethnography, grounded theory and case study is the theoretical stance and design of the research
Methods of data collection and data analysis, including data protection	Non-maleficence	The methods of data collection and analysis need to ensure they do not disrupt the prison regime, or inadvertently capture data on or place a burden on non-participants, or put the security of the prison at risk
Study setting	Beneficence Non-maleficence	Identification of the prison setting and if the research is specific to and can only occur in the prison setting
Sample and eligibility criteria	Autonomy	Inclusiveness of the sample to represent the prison population, including participant from a black, Asian and other minority ethnic background and women prisoners
Sampling, sample size and sampling technique	Justice	An element of sampling that is important in the prison setting is to ensure all eligible prisoners have the opportunity to participate
Recruitment	Autonomy Justice	Recruitment needs to be inclusive to all prisoners, and not biased through the selection of potential participants by prison staff and healthcare professionals
Informed consent and confidentiality	Autonomy	The provision of adequate information, and time to discuss the research to provide an informed decision to participate, if the prisoner has the capacity to make this decision
Research Ethics Committee and regulatory reviews and reports	Autonomy Beneficence Non-maleficence Justice	Detailed information provided in Chapter 7, including a flow diagram or processes

(Continued)

Table 9.1 (Continued)

Component of protocol	Ethical principle	Application
Assessment of risk	Beneficence Non-maleficence	Risk-benefit analysis, emphasis on minimising the risk to prisoners with a focus on the benefits, although equivalence to healthcare and research is not being discussed
Patient and public involvement	Autonomy Beneficence Non-maleficence	Engagement of prisoners, prison staff and other stakeholders in the development of research enables them to be involved in the risk analysis and to ensure the research is acceptable, and the findings and possible recommendations relevant to the needs identified by PPI
Dissemination Policy	Justice	The Final Study Report, and outcomes and recommendations from the research need to be disseminated to all relevant ethics committees and regulatory bodies and to those who participated

Recommendations for further dementia research

A comprehensive programme of research regarding dementia in prison settings is essential. The development of research regarding dementia in the prison setting needs to occur to inform both policy and practice, which address elements at the prisoner/individual level, management/systems, workforce and the environment/setting (Gaston and Axford, 2018):

Prisoner/individual level

- The need to identify appropriate cognitive screening tools for prisoners, and a process of screening for cognitive impairment on admission to prison, and regularly throughout a prison stay
- A cognitive screening process on admission to prison that supports both a possible diagnosis of dementia, and a proactive pathway to support a prisoner with cognitive impairment
- Development of meaningful engagement and purposeful activities, which older prisoners and those with dementia can engage in
- Development of robust method for screening and training programme for prisoners to become 'buddies' and support prisoners with dementia, including training which leads to a recognised certificate/qualification
- Development of a comprehensive approach to a discharge policy to support prisoners with dementia to return to the community and successful resettlement.

Management/systems

- Development of prison reception areas, to support a prisoner with dementia or suspected cognitive impairment when entering the prison setting, and provide a streamlined process and allocation of resources to support these prisoners

- Development of communication and coordination between prison administration and health and social care provision, including the provision of specialist visitors to prison to support prisoners with dementia
- Development of education and training for prison staff, health and social care professionals and fellow prisoners regarding dementia, including signs and symptoms, changes in behaviour and how to support someone with dementia in a prison setting
- Development of a process to provide supervision for prison staff, health and social care professionals and fellow prisoners to be able to debrief and discuss caring for a prisoner with dementia.

Workforce

- Training and education of prison staff, health and social care professionals and prisoners.

Environment / setting

- Modification of a prison setting, and how this is possible in Victorian prisons, in both a timely manner and appropriate for older prisoners and those with dementia.

References

Gaston, S., Axford, A. (2018). Re-framing and re-thinking dementia in the correctional setting. *IntechOpen*, DOI: 0.5772/intechopen.73161.

Lee, C., Haggith, A., Mann, N., Kuhn, I., Carter, F., Eden, B., van Bortel, T. (2016). Older prisoners and the Care Act 2014: an examination of the policy, practice and models of social care delivery. *Prison Service Journal*, 224: 35–41.

Lee, C., Treacy, S., Haggith, A., Darshana, N., Carter, F., Kuhn, I., van Bortel, T. (2019). A systematic integrative review of programmes addressing the social care needs of older prisoners. *Health and Justice*, 7: 9.

Maschi, T., Kwak, J., Ko, E., Morrissey, M.B. (2012). Forget me not: dementia in prison. *The Gerontologist*, 52(4): 441–451.

Prison Reform Trust (2019). *Prison Reform Trust Response to the Justice Committee Inquiry into the Ageing Prison Population*, October. Available from: www.prisonreformtrust.org.uk/Portals/0/Documents/Consultation%20responses/Justice%20Committee%20inquiry%20into%20the%20ageing%20prison%20population.pdf [Accessed on: 12 June 2020].

Index

Page numbers in *italic* indicate a figure and page numbers in **bold** indicate a table on the corresponding page.